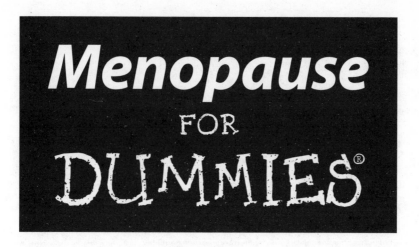

by Marcia L. Jones, PhD

Contributing author Theresa Eichenwald, MD

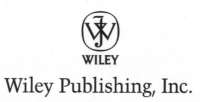

WILEY

Wiley Publishing, Inc.

Menopause For Dummies®

Published by
Wiley Publishing, Inc.
909 Third Avenue
New York, NY 10022
www.wiley.com

Library of Congress Cataloging-in-Publication Data:

Library of Congress Control Number: 2002110330

ISBN: 0-7645-5458-1

Manufactured in the United States of America

10 9 8 7 6 5 4 3 2

1B/RY/RR/QS/IN

About the Authors

Marcia L. Jones, PhD, has life experience in fertility treatment, peri-menopause, and menopause. In 1991, while attempting to start a family at the age of 38, she scoured bookstores searching for down-to-earth information on the likely problems and how to proceed. Her doctor directed her to the only information available at the time, photocopies of technical articles from medical journals and pamphlets written by pharmaceutical companies trying to sell product. Today, many women are delaying childbirth, so the issue of fertility fits nicely into a discussion of perimenopause and menopause. These experiences served as her primary motivation for writing this book. She became certain that women in their mid-thirties to late forties need current, unbiased, reliable information on perimenopause and menopause written for a layperson.

Thanks to the efforts of her doctor Jane Chihal, MD, a contributor to this book and a recognized expert on menopause and fertility, Dr. Jones is the proud mother of two girls ages 6 and 4.

Dr. Jones received her PhD from Southern Methodist University in anthropology. She led many research expeditions in the Middle East and served as an associate professor of anthropology at the University of Tulsa.

Growing weary of academia, Marcia shifted her career focus and entered the fast-paced world of software, achieving the rank of chief operating officer and co-owner of Criterion, a company that developed human-resource software for Fortune 1000 organizations. She grew Criterion from a $1.5 million company to a $10 million company and recently sold it to Peopleclick. During the past 18 years, she has written many articles on people in the workforce and taught courses in the use of human-resource technology as an adjunct professor in the Graduate School of Management at the University of Dallas.

In addition to being the mother of two girls, Marcia just completed her first marathon this past March in Maui and is working on a brown belt in karate.

Contributing author, **Theresa Eichenwald, MD**, has extensive experience caring for menopausal women as an internist at hospitals in New York, Washington D.C., Philadelphia, and, most recently, Texas. She has taught at Albert Einstein School of Medicine and Mount Sinai Medical Center in New York.

In addition to teaching and caring for patients, Dr. Eichenwald has authored a number of articles for professional journals, covering topics such as breast cancer and ovarian tumors as, well as patient education pamphlets. She is a member of the American Medical Association, the American College of Physicians, and in medical school participated in the American Medical Student Association Task Force on Aging.

Dedication

To my father, Dr William S. Jones, Jr., who lit the lamp of curiosity in me, and to my mother, Rebecca Jones, who has supported me through success and failures. My appreciation goes out to my cheering section: Bill Jones, Anne Lee, Barbara Jones, Wendy Fernstrum, William Lewis, Mara Lewis, Becca Lewis, George Lee and Andrew Lee.

To my patient and gracious daughters: Anna Marin Jones and Alexandra Grace Jones. To my ever-faithful partner: Jeannie Caldwell.

Acknowledgments

I am so grateful to the many talented people who have helped create this book. Special thanks to Theresa Eichenwald, MD, for her contributions, collaborations, and review of early versions of this document. Thanks also to her husband Kurt Eichenwald and their three young sons for letting Theresa take the time to author this book.

Acknowledgment is due the Cooper Institute in Dallas for their continuing contributions in the field of preventative medicine.

Thanks to my women friends who insisted that this book was not only needed, but long overdue.

This book would never have gotten to Wiley Publishing if not for Richard and Ginger Simon.

It was a joy working with the wonderful Wiley Publishing staff. These hard-working and talented folks made a tedious editing process seem fun. Special thanks to Natasha Graf, who conceived the idea and encouraged publication of the book. My heartfelt thanks to the guidance and insight of Kathleen Dobie, Project Editor, who tremendously improved the quality of this work. Many thanks to Mike Baker, copy editor, for adding wit and clarity to the text. These folks improved the readability and relevancy of this volume and made sure it was completed on a timely basis. Thanks so much to Kathryn Born, who provided the expressive illustrations that make the text so much more understandable. I am so grateful to Dr. Victoria Ball for her professional reading of the manuscript and expert advice.

Publisher's Acknowledgments

We're proud of this book; please send us your comments through our Dummies online registration form located at www.dummies.com/register/.

Some of the people who helped bring this book to market include the following:

Acquisitions, Editorial, and Media Development

Project Editor: Kathleen A. Dobie

Acquisitions Editor: Natasha Graf

Copy Editor: Mike Baker

Technical Editor: Victoria Ball, MD

Editorial Manager: Christine Meloy Beck

Editorial Assistant: Melissa Bennett

Cover Photos: © Stephen Simpson / Getty Images / FPG

Cartoons: Rich Tennant, www.the5thwave.com

Production

Project Coordinator: Ryan Steffen

Layout and Graphics: Melanie Des Jardins, Tiffany Muth, Jackie Nicholas

Special Art: Kathryn Born

Proofreaders: John Tyler Connoley, Charles Spencer, TECHBOOKS Production Services

Indexer: TECHBOOKS Production Services

Publishing and Editorial for Consumer Dummies

Diane Graves Steele, Vice President and Publisher, Consumer Dummies

Joyce Pepple, Acquisitions Director, Consumer Dummies

Kristin A. Cocks, Product Development Director, Consumer Dummies

Michael Spring, Vice President and Publisher, Travel

Brice Gosnell, Publishing Director, Travel

Suzanne Jannetta, Editorial Director, Travel

Publishing for Technology Dummies

Andy Cummings, Vice President and Publisher, Dummies Technology/General User

Composition Services

Gerry Fahey, Vice President of Production Services

Debbie Stailey, Director of Composition Services

Contents at a Glance

Table of Contents

Introduction

*W*e wrote this book to give women of all ages a clear view of the physical, mental, and emotional changes related to menopause. For generations, women of all ages have wandered blindly into menopause without knowing what to expect. Oh, you probably knew that menopause and hot flashes go hand in hand, but even that information isn't always true. The truth is that you may never have a hot flash, and if you do, it will probably be years before you're menopausal. Common knowledge about menopause is sparse and often wrong. (The medical community didn't even officially recognize the link between estrogen and hot flashes until 1974!)

If menopause only concerned a small group of people on a desert island, this lack of information may be understandable. But over half of the world's population will become menopausal one day. Menopause has been the ugly family member of the research community for years. Even medical textbooks pay scant attention to the topic. Today, one group is paying attention to menopause. The pharmaceutical industry sees great opportunity in the field of menopause, and more research is underway. If you're looking for books to help reasonably intelligent women navigate the jungle of menopause (menopause is uncharted territory), your options are largely limited to pretty, glossy pamphlets published by drug companies (now that's what we call unbiased information) that you can find at your doctor's office. If you're really persistent, you may find some academic articles in medical journals, but your eyes will glass over as you try to pick out straightforward answers to your practical questions. We hope this book can fill that void. Our goal is to help you digest the research so you can make better and objective health decisions.

Menopause is not a medical condition — that's true. No one is going to die from menopause or its symptoms, but every day, women die from the medical effects of low estrogen levels. Your risks of certain diseases and cancers rise after menopause. Some folks may respond to that statement with one of their own, "Well, that's because women are older when they go through menopause." True again, but it's also true that estrogen plays a role in an amazing number of functions in your body, some of which protect your organs, increase your immunity, and slow degeneration. This transformation we call menopause impacts our health in very significant ways. This book helps you understand the story behind the symptoms and the diseases.

Some women choose to use hormone therapy to relieve symptoms associated with menopause and protect their body from disease. The choice of whether to take hormones or not is quite controversial because hormone therapy has its own set of risks. The debate goes on in the medical community and media concerning the risks of hormone therapy. If you're like many women, your confusion only grows as you read more on the subject. Each new study seems to contradict the findings of the last one. You're an intelligent person. But how can you know which study you should believe? In this book, we try to provide enough information to enable you to make informed decisions about your health.

About This Book

We have no agenda in writing this book. We're not trying to sell you medications, alternative health strategies, or remedies. This book presents accurate and up-to-date information from the most credible sources. It contains straightforward information based on reliable medical studies without the academic lingo common to medical journals. When no clear-cut answers exist and when quality research shows mixed conclusions, we let you know.

Everyone's time is limited, so we cut to the chase. We cover the questions that are important to you during this phase of your life. If you want more detail, we provide an appendix full of resources to help with your personal research. We also try not to stray too far from the topic at hand. For example, during the years leading up to menopause, women may have difficulty getting pregnant. The same hormonal changes that cause those annoying symptoms prior to menopause also stifle fertility. Many women in their late thirties who are trying to get pregnant rely on hormone supplements. Despite the overlap in hormonal terms, fertility is not a concern for many women going through the change, so our discussion is limited.

Whether you're going through the change, have already been there, or are about to start off down that road, you'll find the information you need between these snazzy yellow and black covers. We cover all the health issues and therapy choices that confront women during the menopausal years.

Foolish Assumptions

Every author has to make a few assumptions about her audience, and we've made a few assumptions about you:

- ✔ You're a woman. (Sorry, guys, but menopause is a girls-only club.)
- ✔ You want to understand what's going on with your body.

✔ You're looking for straight talk for real people as opposed to scientific jargon and Medicalese (though we have a Medicalese icon to warn you when we stray into this territory).

✔ You want to evaluate your risks of disease as you pass through midlife and move into your menopausal years.

✔ You don't want a book that claims to let you diagnose yourself or figure out what medications you need. You have a medical advisor to discuss these things with.

✔ You want to be able to ask intelligent questions and discuss treatment alternatives with your healthcare providers.

✔ You want to feel more confident about the quality of your healthcare.

✔ You buy every book that has a black and yellow cover.

If any of these statements apply to you, you're in the right place.

How This Book Is Organized

We've organized this book into five parts so you can go directly to the topic that interests you the most. Here's a brief overview of each part:

Part 1: The Main Facts about Menopause

The journey to menopause often catches women by surprise. You may not have been expecting to take the journey, or you may have been wondering when you would begin. In this part, we give you a quick overview of what your hormones are doing before, during, and after menopause. If you haven't thought about things like hormones and follicles for a while, don't worry; we refresh your memory. Your sixth-grade health-and-hygiene course probably never finished the story. In this part, you get the whole story from how the egg makes its journey from the ovary to the uterus to what happens when the ovary goes into retirement.

Part II: The Effects of Menopause on Your Body and Mind

Want to know how hormones affect the health of your body and mind? You can find the answers in Part II. We devote each chapter in this part to a specific body part or health issue. In each chapter, you get an overview of how hormones function in relation to this part of your body and the types of conditions that can develop, how to recognize them, and what you can do about them.

Part III: Treating the Effects

You may want to evaluate the pros and cons of hormone therapy (HT) from time to time during your journey through menopause. This part of the book brings you up to date on what the medical community knows about HT. We discuss the effects of HT so that you can make informed decisions. Reading these chapters provides added benefits as well: You'll probably find it easier to evaluate the news about hormone research that comes out in future years.

We also include information about non-HT drugs and alternative treatments.

Part IV: Lifestyle Issues for Menopause and Beyond

Part IV is chock full of great ways to stay healthy and enjoy a long and active life during and after menopause. Staying healthy and active is simpler than you think. We discuss healthy eating habits and simple ways to stay fit. Whether you're looking for natural ways to lower your risk of specific diseases or for ways to slow the aging process, you can find the information you need right here.

Part V: The Part of Tens

If you're a fan of *For Dummies* books, you probably recognize this part. These are short chapters with quick tips and fast facts. In Part V, we debunk ten menopause myths, review ten common medical tests you may encounter, and suggest ten terrific exercise programs for menopausal women.

Part VI: Appendixes

A glossary of menopause-related terms and a list of menopause-related resources cap the book.

Conventions Used in This Book

We use our own brand of shorthand for some frequently used terms, and icons to highlight specific information. The following sections help you get used to these conventions.

Taking in shorthand

As you read this book, you'll discover that menopause is a process, with different stages characterized by similar symptoms. These stages are referred to as *perimenopause,* the 3 to 10 years prior to menopause when you may experience symptoms; *menopause* itself, which you know you've reached only after you've reached it because the definition of menopause is the absence of periods for a year; and *postmenopause,* which is your life after you've stopped having periods. In this book, we use *perimenopause* to describe the premenopause condition, and we use *menopause* to refer to everything after that just because the term *postmenopause* isn't commonly used.

A major part of this book — the whole of Part III as well as sections in other chapters — talks about hormone therapy (HT), which is used to alleviate symptoms and address health concerns prompted by menopause. In literature and on Web sites, you can see hormone therapies referred to and abbreviated any number of ways, including hormone replacement therapy (HRT) and estrogen replacement therapy (ERT). But we stick pretty closely to using HT because we feel that it's the most inclusive and accurate term. Just be aware that *HT* means essentially the same thing as *HRT.*

And, speaking of hormones, a couple of the more important ones for menopausal women have several subcategories:

- Types of **estrogen** include estriol, estradiol, and estrone.
- **Progesterone** is the class of hormone; the form used in hormone therapy is often referred to as progestin.

We sometimes use these terms interchangeably and only refer to the specific hormone as necessary for clarity.

Eyeing the icons

In this book, we use icons as a quick way to go directly to the information you need. Look for the icons in the margin that point out specific types of information. Here's what the icons we use in this book mean.

The Tip icon points out practical, concise information that can help you take better care of yourself.

This icon points you to medical terms and jargon that can help you understand what you read or hear from professionals and enable you to ask your healthcare provider intelligent questions.

This fine piece of art flags information that's worth noting.

When you see this icon, do what it tells you to do. It accompanies info that should be discussed with an expert in the field.

The Technical Stuff icon points out material that generally can be classified as dry as a bone. Although we think that the information is interesting, it's not vital to your understanding of the issue. Skip it if you so desire.

This icon cautions you about potential problems or threats to your health.

Where to Go from Here

For Dummies books are designed so that you can dip in anywhere that looks interesting and get the information you need. This is a reference book, so don't feel like you have to read an entire chapter (or even an entire section for that matter). You won't miss anything by skipping around. So, find what interests you and jump on in!

Part I
The Main Facts about Menopause

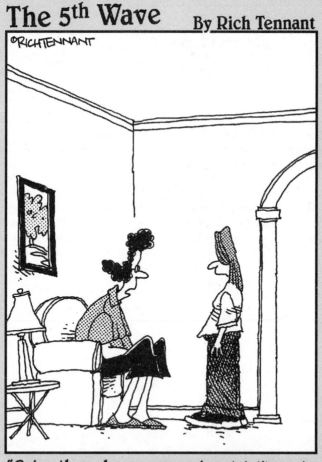

The 5th Wave   By Rich Tennant

"Going through menopause is a lot like going through adolescence, but no, I'm not in love with Justin Timberlake, I don't hate your little brother, and I have no desire to dye my hair green."

In this part . . .

*T*he first act of *Dance of the Hormones* probably occurred three decades or so ago for you. You remember that one don't you? The bittersweet tale of teenage angst and joy that we call puberty. And now, intermission (the menstrual years) may be coming to a close as the hormones once again take the stage for the second act — menopause. Well, take your seat and get ready to peruse your program . . . uh, Part I of this book.

In Part I, we provide you with an outline to your menopausal years. We define menopause, review the biology, introduce you to the actors — your hormones — and briefly review the related symptoms and health conditions (physical, mental, and emotional). Get to it before the usher dims the lights.

Chapter 1

Reversing Puberty

· ·

· ·

"*Y*ou've come a long way, baby" seems like a recurring slogan for baby boomers. The phrase certainly says a lot about the women of this generation as they approach the rite of passage we call menopause. As an individual, you no doubt feel like you've come a long way in your life by the time you begin to think about menopause. Society, in general, and women, in particular, have also come a long way in opening up the discussion about the mysteries of menopause.

Puberty and menopause bracket the reproductive season of your life, and they share many characteristics. Both puberty and menopause are transitions (meaning that they don't last forever), they're both triggered by hormones, and they both cause physical and emotional changes (that sometimes drive you crazy).

Puberty was the time when your hormones first swung into action. It marked the beginning of your reproductive years. Remember the ride? Your hormone levels shifted wildly and caused your first menstrual period. And don't forget the erratic emotions — what we like to call the teenage crazies. Over the course of a few years, your hormones found a comfortable level. Your unpredictable periods finally settled into a predictable pattern, and your emotional balance was more or less restored.

At the end of your reproductive years, your hormone levels go through a similar dance (this time causing the midlife crazies), but your hormones eventually find a new, lower level of production. Your periods are erratic for a while, but they eventually wind down and stop. Just in case you're wondering, those midlife emotional crazies eventually pass too.

Keep in mind that the phrase "you've come a long way, baby" closes with "but you've got such a long way to go." Women today often live 40 or 50 years after menopause. We all want to enjoy these years by visiting friends, taking care of our loved ones and ourselves, and continuing to participate in activities that give us pleasure.

In this chapter, we introduce you to menopause so you know what to expect when the time comes or what has been happening to you if you're already in transition.

Defining Menopause

Have you ever noticed how you don't really pay close attention to directions or where you're going when you're the passenger in a car? You only start to worry about every exit number and stop light when you're the one behind the wheel. Well, menopause is like that. We all hear about menopause and menopausal symptoms, but we rarely pay much attention to the particulars until it's our turn.

When you do slide into the driver's seat and start paying attention, you may become frustrated by the confusing terminology associated with the whole menopause thing. Aside from the pamphlets you get from the doctor's office, most books, magazines, and articles treat menopause like a stage that starts with hot flashes and goes on for the rest of your life. But, *menopause* actually means the end of menstruation. During the years leading up to menopause (called *perimenopause*), your periods may be so erratic that you're never sure which period will be the last one, but you aren't officially menopausal until you haven't had a period for a year.

A lot happens *before* you have your last period, and all this physical and mental commotion is associated with menopause. You may experience hot flashes, mental lapses, mood swings, and heart palpitations while you're still having periods. But, when you ask your doctor if you're menopausal, he or she may check you over and say "no." Relax: Your doctor isn't wrong, and you aren't crazy. You're not menopausal. You're *peri*menopausal.

Medical folks divide menopause into phases that coincide with physiological changes. We describe these phases in just a second, but you need to know something about the terminology that surrounds menopause. On one hand, you have the medical terms associated with menopause, and on the other, you have the terms that you hear when you're chatting with the girls over coffee or tennis.

The term *perimenopause* refers to the time leading up to the cessation of menstruation, when estrogen production is slowing down. A lot of the symptoms that folks usually label as *menopausal* (hot flashes, mood swings, sleeplessness, and so on) actually take place during the perimenopausal years. We're sticklers in this book about using the term *perimenopause* rather than *menopause* to describe this early phase because you're still having periods. We also use *perimenopause* because we want to note the physiological and emotional changes you experience prior to the end of your periods and distinguish them from the changes that happen after your body has adjusted to lower levels of estrogen.

Technically, the time after your last period is called *postmenopause,* but this word has never really caught on. So, in keeping with common usage, we most often use the term *menopause* to refer to the actual event and the years after menopause and use *postmenopause* only when it helps clarify things. When we talk about *menopausal* women in this book, we're talking about women who have stopped having periods — whether they're 55 or 75.

The years leading up to and following menopause mark a pretty major transformation in a woman's life. As you make your way through this period of your life, you'll want to know where you're at within the whole grand scope of the change and what's going on inside you. Here's a brief description of the phases associated with menopause. (Don't worry: We give you a lot more detail about the various stages in other chapters.)

Making changes while approaching the change: Perimenopause

Perimenopause is the stage during which your hormones start to change gears. Some months, your hormones operate at the levels they've worked at for the past 30 years or so; other months, your ovaries are tired and don't produce estrogen when they should. Your brain responds to this lack of estrogen production by sending a signal to try to get those ovaries jumpstarted. When they receive the signal, your ovaries leap out of bed and overcompensate for their laziness by producing double or triple the normal amount of estrogen.

Your period is late because your ovaries were dozing during the first part of your normal cycle. Your period is super heavy because, when your ovaries wake up, they overcompensate by producing way too much estrogen. (Just like you may run around like a chicken with its head cut off after you wake up having slept through your alarm.)

So, during perimenopause, you still have your period, but you experience symptoms that folks associate with menopause. If you go to the doctor at this stage and ask, "What's happening to me? Could this be menopause?" the doctor will often go straight to the "Could this be menopause?" part of your question. Of course you're not menopausal if you're still having periods. But the problem is that many doctors miss the first part of the question — the "What's happening to me?" part. This is the real issue you want to get to the bottom of — the cause of your weird physical and emotional conditions.

Menstruating no more: To menopause and beyond

Menopause means never having to say, "Can I borrow a tampon," again.

If you haven't had a period for a year, you've reached *menopause*. Women can become menopausal approximately anytime between the ages of 45 and 55, with the average age being 51. The definition may seem cut and dry at first glance, but here are a few situations that may leave you scratching your head.

What if you use a cyclical type of hormone therapy in which you take estrogen for several days and progestin during the last few days of your cycle? You still have a period (the progestin causes you to slough the lining of the uterus), but you don't ovulate. Are you menopausal or not? Technically, you're delaying your last period. You're taking a sufficient dosage of estrogen to rid yourself of perimenopausal symptoms, but you're no longer fertile.

Here's another tricky one: If you've had a *hysterectomy* (surgical removal of the uterus), you're menopausal according to the basic definition. But, if you had your uterus removed but kept your ovaries, you're not "hormonally" menopausal because your ovaries still produce estrogen. By taking your blood and analyzing your hormone levels, your physician can tell you whether your hormones are officially at menopausal levels.

These tricky situations cause us to ask, "Who cares about the definition?" You know a rose is a rose. The main concern here is *what's happening with your hormones,* especially estrogen. Hormonal changes can trigger many physical and emotional health issues.

When you reach menopause, your hormone production is so low that your periods stop. Your ovaries still produce some estrogen and testosterone, but instead of producing hormones in cycles (which is why you have periods and why you're only fertile for about four or five days each month), your body now produces constant, low levels of hormones. The type of estrogen your ovaries churn out also switches from an active type to a rather inactive form.

Postmenopause is the period of your life that starts after menopause (a year after your last period) and ends when you do. This is a time when your body is living on greatly reduced levels of estrogen, testosterone, and progesterone. In this book, we simply refer to both the cessation of your period and your life afterwards as menopause.

Anticipating Menopause

When will you become menopausal? The timing varies from woman to woman. Predicting this stuff is nowhere near an exact science. Heck, you can't even use the fact that you started your period earlier than most women as a predictor that you'll stop menstruating earlier. (The same goes for starting your period later in life and ending it later in life.) Genetics and lifestyle may have some impact on the schedule, but basically, it happens when it happens. But we can give you some ballpark age ranges for these phases.

Most women become perimenopausal sometime between the ages of 35 and 50. You'll probably know it when you get there because you'll probably have some of the symptoms (check out the Cheat Sheet at the front of this book and Chapter 3) and/or some irregular periods. Women usually become menopausal sometime in their fifties.

Some events can alter these "normal" age patterns, including lifestyle habits and medical interventions. Here are a few exceptional types of menopause:

- **Premature menopause:** A term used when women go through menopause in their thirties. This timing is considered unusually early, but it may be normal for you.

- **Medical menopause:** Refers to menopause induced by chemotherapy or radiation therapy. Sometimes these treatments can cause a pause in your body's normal cycle. However, this type of menopause is often reversed after treatments are finished, though your periods may take a month, several months, or even years to return.

- **Surgical menopause:** Refers to menopause induced by surgery. Removal of both ovaries results in immediate, nonreversible menopause.

  Because your ovaries produce all types of sex hormones (estrogen, progesterone, and testosterone), surgical removal of your ovaries is fairly traumatic for your system, and you typically experience intense perimenopausal symptoms (hot flashes and the like).

Excessive exercising or an eating disorder can cause a temporary halt in your periods (a condition called *amenorrhea*), but your periods will return to normal when your lifestyle returns to normal. This is not menopause but rather a medical condition that needs to be treated.

Men-o-pause

When men experience mood swings and mental lapses during their fifties, they (or you) may think that they're going through the change too. But the change men go through is quite different from the one women experience.

The rise and fall of hormones in a woman's body follows a cyclical pattern. Hormone levels shift throughout the month on a regular basis. So, every 28 to 35 days, a woman has the chance to become pregnant. The hormonal changes prepare her body for conception and pregnancy.

Men have no cycle (besides, perhaps, the yearly cycle based on the presence or absence of football in their systems). Their primary sex hormone, testosterone, stays at a fairly constant level from day to day, so men don't experience cyclical fluctuations. But men's testosterone levels do decline with age. Lower testosterone levels generally result in lower libido (sex drive) in males and generally occur when men are in their late fifties or sixties.

Do men go through menopause? There's no question that the decline of sex hormones in men results in lower libido, weaker bones, and an increased risk of prostate cancer. But the changes are simply a result of the natural aging process and are not triggered by a change in hormonal patterns.

Experiencing Menopause

When a group of women talk about their personal experiences of puberty, menstrual cycles, and pregnancy, the stories are all over the board. Some women don't notice changes in their bodies; others recognize the moment ovulation or conception occurs. Some women have terrible problems with premenstrual syndrome (PMS); others have trouble-free cycles throughout their entire lives. Women's experiences vary with perimenopause and menopause just as much as they vary with these other changes.

Identifying symptoms

We devote Chapter 3 almost exclusively to the symptoms women may experience during perimenopause. Several other chapters explain the link between your hormones and these symptoms.

Less than half of all women experience annoying symptoms such as hot flashes, heart palpitations, interrupted sleep, and mood swings during the transition period prior to menopause. Most women who do experience these symptoms experience the symptoms while they're still menstruating on a regular schedule.

Other women recognize that they're perimenopausal because their periods, which used to be as regular as clockwork, are now irregular. Their periods may be late, they may skip a period, or their flow may be light one month and resemble a flood the next month.

Unfortunately no objective medical test exists to determine whether you're officially perimenopausal.

Calling in the professionals

If you're in your late forties or fifties and you're experiencing the symptoms listed on the Cheat Sheet and in Chapter 3, you can probably assume that you're perimenopausal. But don't cancel that appointment with your medical advisor to get the symptoms checked out. (If you don't have an appointment to cancel, make one and keep it.) Many symptoms of perimenopause are the same as some of the symptoms of thyroid problems, cardiovascular disease, depression, and other serious health issues.

Your medical practitioner can help you deal with the undesirable symptoms of perimenopause and prevent serious health conditions that are more prevalent after menopause.

Making Time for Menopause

You may be wondering when the perimenopause and menopause phase of your life will hit and how long the symptoms will last.

Starting out

Most women's ovaries begin a transformation sometime between the ages of 35 and 50. If you start the change before you reach 40, you experience what's known as *premature menopause.*

Perimenopause is sometimes called a climacteric period, which simply means that it's a crucial period. Remember that your ovaries don't just shut down one day; the transition is punctuated with production peaks and valleys that cause many annoying physical and mental symptoms. Perimenopause is a time of important physiological change — when egg production slows along with the production of estrogen and progesterone begins slowing down.

Seeing it through to the end

Because you never really know when perimenopause starts, accurately defining a timeframe is difficult. Some women experience symptoms for ten years before their periods stop. The fact is that most of the symptoms you hear about are caused by the fluctuating hormone levels of perimenopause as opposed to the sustained, low levels of hormones you experience during menopause.

You're officially menopausal one year after your last period. After that, many people use the term postmenopause to mark the rest of your life (though in this book, we just keep using *menopause*).

Treating Menopause

At the end of the perimenopause road, your ovaries (and consequently, your hormone production) finally wind down. Your body gradually adjusts to the lower hormone levels typical of life after menopause. Most of the peri-menopausal symptoms disappear, but now your concerns shift to health issues associated with prolonged, lowered levels of active estrogen.

Estrogen not only plays a role in reproduction, it also helps regulate a host of other functions throughout your body. Estrogen protects your bones and cardiovascular system, among other responsibilities. Those pesky peri-menopausal symptoms may make life miserable, but they aren't dangerous to your health. But the conditions associated with long periods of diminished estrogen levels are very troublesome. They include

- ✔ Cardiovascular disease
- ✔ Heart disease
- ✔ Hypertension (high blood pressure)
- ✔ Osteoporosis
- ✔ Stroke

So you and your doctor need to work on strategies to prevent these conditions.

Some women choose hormone therapy (HT) to help prevent disease; others choose to take medications as individual problems arise. (We cover hormone therapy in Chapters 10 through 15 and non-hormonal ways to deal with certain conditions in Chapters 17.) Some women try alternatives to traditional medicine such as herbs or acupuncture (check out Chapter 16). Whichever path or paths you choose, each strategy presents benefits and risks. Your choices depend on your medical history, your family history, and your healthcare preferences. And remember that both your experiences and medical technologies change daily, so re-evaluate your options from time to time.

Promoting Longevity

Not long ago, 50 was about as old as we could expect to get. Today, many of us will live well into our seventies, eighties, and nineties. The fact that most women stop being fertile in their forties doesn't mean that women are no longer productive after 40. In fact, with the whole reproduction thing out of the way, women have more time and opportunities to make new contributions to life on earth (or in space).

One of the keys to a long and happy life is good genes. Another key is taking good care of yourself and the genes you're dealt. Regular checkups can address medical issues as they arise and help prevent others. Eat healthy foods (and portions), get some exercise, and live life to its fullest.

Everyone agrees that a healthy lifestyle is the best way to reduce troublesome perimenopausal symptoms, prevent disease, and promote a long and healthy life. It's also the least risky strategy for dealing with perimenopause and menopause. Taking up this challenge requires self-assessment and a bit of determination. Shifting to a healthy lifestyle involves eliminating unhealthy habits, getting at least a half-hour of aerobic exercise five times a week, and maintaining a healthy, balanced diet that includes at least five servings of fruit and vegetables each week. We provide some great info on diet, nutrition, and exercise in Chapters 18 and 19.

Chapter 2

Talking Biology and Psychology: Your Mind and Body on Menopause

● ●

In This Chapter

▶ Reviewing the menstrual cycle

▶ Getting to know your sex hormones

▶ Mapping out the stages of menopause

● ●

*I*f you're in your forties, and you're like a lot women, you've asked your-self, "What in the world is happening to me?" Maybe that persistent ring of fat around your waist brings the question to mind. You know what we're talking about — that extra girth that seemingly appeared overnight and now won't go away no matter how many crunches you do. Or maybe you notice yourself perspiring while lying in bed next to your partner just like you did when you first got together — except now it happens in the middle of the night when you're not even thinking about *that*. Does it seem as if the world has gotten dumber and that no one can do things right anymore? Maybe it's not the new millennium that's causing your irritability and mood swings, maybe it's perimenopause.

In this chapter, we take a look at how your hormones work during your reproductive years and how they change as you approach and enter your nonreproductive years. The physiological, emotional, and mental changes you may notice during perimenopause and menopause are largely triggered by fluctuations or deviations in your hormone levels.

Setting the Stage

Before we get started, we need to set the stage. Menopause is a natural and necessary change in life; it's not a disease, deficiency, or failure.

You may see and hear medical terms such as *estrogen deficiency, ovarian failure,* and *vaginal atrophy* used to describe menopause and its symptoms — most of them in this book. These terms aren't meant to carry negative connotations. They're meant to describe expected conditions. Viewing menopause as a natural change — not an organ failure — is important.

Your ovaries live a double life — one as the holder of the seeds of life (*oocytes* that later develop into eggs), and the other as a maintenance worker. Menopause marks the shift from the first life to the second life. No longer busy with developing follicles that carry eggs (which release lots of estrogen), the ovaries move onto the methodical production of low levels of hormones to maintain body functions.

Just as women aren't put on earth for the simple purpose of bearing children, your ovaries aren't there just to supply eggs. Your ovaries are a critical source of hormones for your body, and they continue to produce hormones well after menopause (in much smaller amounts than before). Your ovaries don't retire; they experience a career change.

Because the life expectancy for most people in the United States is about 80 years, the average woman spends a little more than half her life menstruating and being fertile. Therefore, you can expect to spend a significant portion of your life just being a woman — not going through puberty or menopause or the periods in between.

Medical professionals who view menopause as a natural change focus less on trying to "fix a failure" and more on preventing future health issues.

In some circles, the administration of hormone therapy (HT) has the reputation of being a part of the fix-a-failure approach to menopause. But a growing body of research shows that HT can help prevent, postpone, or treat a number of health issues that threaten menopausal women.

Making the Menstrual Cycle and Hormone Connection

Okay, admit it. You didn't actually pay attention to those long, boring, sterile movies that explained menstruation to you and your sixth-grade classmates.

You know the ones — the health-class movies with titles like "You're a Woman Now." (Back in those days, we didn't have interesting titles like *Sex For Dummies*.) If you were anything like us, you had difficulty making the connection between the two-dimensional, black-and-white illustrations of female organs and the three-dimensional, high-definition experiences of bloating and cramps.

In this section, we make the connection between your sex hormones and your lifelong menstrual cycle (hopefully in a much clearer and more meaningful fashion than those old movies made it).

One of the major functions of sex hormones is to prepare the body to produce life. So visiting your sex hormones at the reproduction office to watch them do their jobs as a team is a good place to start the discussion. Then we take a closer look at each individual member of Team Hormone.

The average menstrual cycle is 28 days, but a cycle that lasts anywhere from 22 to 35 days is normal. For the purpose of this discussion, we use a 28-day cycle; you can adjust the numbers as necessary to fit your personal calendar. Figure 2-1 shows hormone levels throughout a menstrual cycle.

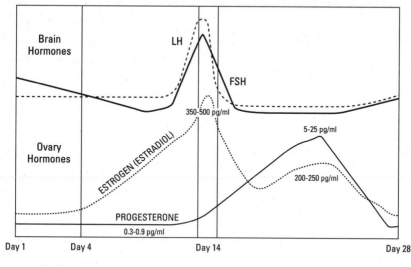

Figure 2-1: Hormone levels throughout the menstrual cycle.

Day 1 of your cycle is the first day of your period (see the "Days of our lives: Determining Day 1" sidebar for help determining the first day of your period). Your body begins flushing out the lining of your uterus, which isn't needed because a fertilized egg requiring nourishment and support isn't present in your uterus.

Days of our lives: Determining Day 1

The first day of your period is called Day 1. Simple enough, huh? Sounds pretty definitive. Well, maybe not. When it comes to your body, nothing is ever truly definitive. Here's how things can get a bit more complicated: Do you count yesterday as Day 1 because you had some light bleeding? Or do you call today Day 1 because you really started flowing today? Or maybe you should count two days ago as Day 1 because you started cramping really badly and had a bit of spotting.

How to solve this dilemma? Consistency is key. If you normally have a light day before you start your regular flow, count your light day as Day 1. But, if you're like some women who experience spotting several days before they actually begin their period, Day 1 should be the first day of your regular flow.

Your ovaries are filled with little seeds (eggs) surrounded by support cells (*stroma*). During the first half of your cycle (Days 1 to 14), hormones produced in your brain — *follicle-stimulating hormone* (FSH) and *luteinizing hormone* (LH) — and hormones produced in your ovaries — estrogen — work together to develop and then release an egg. (For more information on FSH and LH see the "Heading up your hormones" section later in this chapter.) During these first two weeks, your estradiol estrogen levels are on the rise, and your progesterone levels are very low. This particular hormone combination (high estrogen, low progesterone) is why you usually feel so good during this stretch of your cycle. You owe your energy, restful sleep, upbeat mood, sharp memory, and terrific concentration to your old friend, estrogen, which plays a role in many physical and mental systems — not just your reproductive system.

As soon as the brain senses that estrogen levels are right, it produces a surge of luteinizing hormone (LH), which triggers the release of an egg — otherwise known as *ovulation*. Ovulation usually occurs between Day 12 and Day 16 of your cycle. (You want the scoop on LH? Check out the "Heading up your hormones" section later in this chapter.)

After you've ovulated, estrogen levels drop, and progesterone production kicks in. *Progesterone,* which peaks around Day 20, is a hormone that gets the uterus ready for a baby. If the egg is fertilized, your progesterone levels stay high. If the egg isn't fertilized, progesterone and estrogen levels drop and menstruation occurs.

Surveying the Role of Hormones

Unless you're a gynecologist, you may not be able to remember what all of the hormones do (or what the crazy abbreviations stand for). So we've included

Table 2-1 as a quick review of all the specifics on the operative hormones and their functions.

Table 2-1		Hormones in a Nutshell
Hormone	*Produced By*	*Main Activities*
Estrogens	Ovaries	Female hormones that promote breast development and cause menstrual cycles, ovulation, pregnancy, and more.
Estrone (E1)		An "inactive" form of estrogen. After menopause, estrone is the dominant form of estrogen in your body. It's produced in the ovaries prior to menopause. After menopause, body fat produces estrone. High levels of estrone may be associated with breast and endometrial cancer.
Estradiol (E2)		The "active" form of estrogen produced mainly in the ovaries. Services hundreds of mental and physical functions in a woman's body. Prior to menopause, it's the dominant form of estrogen in your body.
Estriol (E3)		Form of estrogen only found in pregnant women.
Follicle-stimulating hormone (FSH)	Pituitary gland	Hormone produced in the brain that stimulates the ovaries to get follicles growing and producing estrogen. This is the hormone that kicks off the ovulation cycle.
Luteinizing hormone (LH)	Pituitary gland	Hormone produced in the brain that triggers the follicle to release the egg (ovulation). LH supports the production of estrogen and progesterone by the abandoned egg sac known as the *corpus luteum.*
Progesterone	Ovaries	Prepares the womb for pregnancy and helps maintain pregnancy. While estrogen is the dominant hormone in the first half of your menstrual cycle, progesterone is dominant in the second half. The effects of progesterone also include water retention, sweet cravings, and fatigue. High doses can work as a sedative or as a depressant. The synthetic form of progesterone is called *progestin.*

(continued)

Table 2-1 *(continued)*		
Hormone	**Produced By**	**Main Activities**
Testosterone	Ovaries	Considered a "male hormone" even though the bodies of both men and women produce it. In women, the ovaries produce it. During the change, testosterone levels drop. Testosterone benefits women by maintaining healthy libido, strong bones, and muscle growth.

Heading up your hormones

Your brain produces the hormones that direct the production of sex hormones in your ovaries. You might say that the hormones produced by your brain act as senior management, directing operations in your ovaries. The hormones in your ovaries are the field managers, directing operations in the field, which is your entire body. The hormones produced by your brain include

- ✓ **Follicle-stimulating hormone (FSH):** When the brain senses that estrogen and progesterone levels have dropped, it shoots out some FSH to the ovaries to tell them to begin developing *follicles* (nutritious sacs that cover the eggs) and start producing estrogen.

- ✓ **Luteinizing hormone (LH):** This hormone triggers ovulation. When LH surges, the follicle releases the egg. The abandoned follicle wrapping, the *corpus luteum,* secretes progesterone and estrogen.

Explaining estrogen

Oh how very sophisticated women are. We don't just produce estrogen; we produce three different types of estrogen:

- ✓ **Estradiol:** Active estrogen
- ✓ **Estrone:** Inactive estrogen predominant after menopause
- ✓ **Estriol:** Estrogen produced only during pregnancy

Medical folks use a shorthand system when speaking about estrogen to avoid confusion (and lengthy sentences). They refer to estrone as E1, estradiol as E2, and estriol as E3.

Throughout the book, we use the generic term *estrogen* to mean all the different types of estrogen, unless distinguishing among them is important for the discussion at hand.

Estradiol (E2)

You may hear doctors or nurses refer to estradiol by its scientific name, *17-beta estradiol,* but most folks know it as "the good stuff." Before menopause, estradiol is the predominant form of estrogen produced by your ovaries and used throughout your body. Estradiol actively helps out with hundreds of different physical and mental functions.

After menopause, your ovaries stop producing estradiol, and that's when you develop many of those annoying symptoms such as hot flashes, palpitations, changes in your skin, bone, hair, and blood vessels, headaches, and so on.

Your body can convert estrone to estradiol but only with fully functioning ovaries. Your ovaries are slowing down during perimenopause and menopause, and your body doesn't get nearly as much estradiol after menopause as it was used to during your reproductive years.

Estrone (E1)

After menopause, estrone is the predominant type of estrogen streaming through your body. Estrone is made by your body fat and, before menopause, by your ovaries. The more body fat you have, the more estrone you have. Estrone is mainly a stored form of estrogen. Prior to menopause, your ovaries can convert estrone to the active form of estrogen, estradiol. That conversion only happens in premenopausal ovaries.

Estriol (E3)

The weakest of the three estrogens is estriol, which your placenta produces only if you're pregnant. If you don't have any estriol in your body, it's okay; it just means you aren't pregnant.

Promoting progesterone

If all these hormone names are confusing to you, here's a tip that can help you make sense of progesterone. Think of progesterone as *pro*moting *gest*ation; it prepares your womb to nurture a fertilized egg.

Most of your progesterone is made after ovulation. If your egg is fertilized, the placenta takes over progesterone production during the eighth or ninth week of pregnancy. If the egg isn't fertilized, progesterone levels drop. This lack of progesterone triggers your period. Many doctors believe that symptoms of premenstrual syndrome (PMS) can be attributed to progesterone. You can thank progesterone when you crave sweets, feel fatigued, retain water, and develop acne.

Progesterone gets your body ready to support a pregnancy. How does this play out? When progesterone levels are high, you feel hungry more often.

Progesterone also slows down the digestion process so that you can absorb nutrients better, but that slower digestion process can make you feel bloated or constipated.

Progesterone can cause depression and increase your cholesterol levels. Progesterone also has a sedating effect that makes some women feel calm and others feel lethargic. It's all a matter of perception, but it isn't your imagination. Progesterone has been found to be eight times more potent than one of the drugs used in anesthesia!

Investigating androgens

Yes, Virginia, your body does produce "male" hormones, and it's perfectly normal. Both men and (to a lesser degree) women produce a group of hormones called androgens in their adrenal glands and sex organs (testes in men, ovaries in women). The androgens affected by menopause are testosterone and DHEA.

As you age, your body slows its production of both female and male hormones. During the transition of menopause, estrogen and androgen levels can get a bit out of balance. Even though your androgen levels typically decrease as estrogen levels decrease, the big decrease in estrogen levels can alter the balance so that androgen has a greater relative presence than it did before menopause. This imbalance leads to changes:

- Fat migrates toward your waist.
- Hair disappears from your head and starts growing on your chin or upper lip.
- Blood pressure rises.
- Total cholesterol rises.

Okay, okay. Stop cursing your androgens already. They have many positive effects on women's bodies too. Check it out:

- **Testosterone:** This hormone triggers sexual desire. That's right — testosterone promotes a healthy sexual desire in women. Testosterone also helps women build bone, maintain muscle mass (so you burn fat), and maintain optimal energy levels.
- **DHEA:** First an introduction is in order. *DHEA* stands for *dehydroepiandrosterone* (that's why we use the abbreviation). DHEA is a building block for testosterone. Your ovaries covert the DHEA from your adrenal glands into testosterone. Without DHEA you could forget about all those positives associated with testosterone.

This building-block hormone is available in over-the-counter form and can cause unwanted side effects if you're not careful. Conversion of DHEA to testosterone requires functioning ovaries. During perimenopause and beyond, your ovaries aren't peak performers. Also, the benefits of testosterone and DHEA can't be achieved without the presence of estradiol. Because DHEA is unregulated, you may not know how much you need or how much you're getting. So, if you're going to use DHEA, use it under the watchful eye of a healthcare professional.

Acting Out the Stages of Menopause

Menopause, the permanent pause in your periods (*menses*), is one of those things that you aren't sure happened until long after it's over. Like the first time you met your best friend: You probably had no idea that you'd become so close. You only realized how special that occasion really was when you were able to look back on it. Okay, maybe menopause isn't a warm-and-fuzzy-greeting-card occasion, but it is a passage worth noting.

Are you or aren't you menopausal? You can answer that question only after the fact — after you've gone a year without your period. Many of the annoying symptoms assigned to menopause actually are much worse prior to menopause in the phase known as *perimenopause.* During perimenopause, you get both the annoying symptoms (hot flashes, irritability, mood swings, and so on) and your period. Lucky you.

In this section, we clarify what's happening to your body during the various stages of menopause and tell you how to recognize where you are in the great transition.

Previewing perimenopause

For most women, perimenopause is a big case of déjà vu. Remember puberty (vaguely)? Remember the crying jags, the mood swings, and the "what's wrong with my skin!" traumas? Well, guess what? They're b-a-a-a-ck. Once again your hormones are ready to wreak havoc on your body, your emotions, and your mental faculties. This time around, however, you're a bit wiser (you bought this book, didn't you?), you have experience dealing with change, and you realize that this too shall pass.

To this day, some doctors advise women who are still experiencing periods not to worry about "menopausal" symptoms. But you know (because you read it here) that the symptoms folks often attribute to menopause are usually felt as intensely or more intensely during perimenopause. And perimenopause can last for ten years before a woman stops menstruating altogether and becomes truly menopausal.

Periodic periods

During perimenopause, things change. If you welcomed your period on the same day as the full moon for 20 years, you may wake up to find the planets suddenly out of alignment.

The hormonal shift is due to changes happening in your ovaries. Your ovaries hold little *oocytes* (seeds), and each month, some of these seeds develop into *follicles* (little sacs that hold an egg). One or two lucky follicles mature and release an egg. That's when you ovulate. The oocytes in your ovaries are held together by a substance called *stroma.* The stroma produce testosterone, and the follicles produce estrogen. When you're very young, you have hundreds of thousands of these little seeds. As you age, you have fewer seeds and more stroma. As the mix of seeds and stroma in your ovaries changes, so does hormone production. Your ovaries decrease their production of estrogen but continue to produce testosterone.

Sometimes you ovulate during your cycle; sometimes you don't. Sometimes the FSH just doesn't get the follicles producing estrogen right off the bat. Estrogen levels are low at the beginning of your cycle when they should be high. Your brain responds to this lack of get-up-and-go by sending another surge of FSH (see the "Heading up your hormones" section earlier in this chapter). Finally getting the message, your ovaries become a little frantic and go into double-time production of estrogen. Right at the time when you should be ovulating and producing progesterone, your ovaries are just kicking into gear developing a follicle. That means you won't ovulate when you usually do and your period will be late.

Your menstrual cycle is all messed up. Your estrogen shoots up, and then it drops down. You get hot flashes and maybe even heart palpitations (a racing heart) when estrogen plunges. But just when you're convinced that something is funny and you need to schedule a doctor's appointment, you get your period and everything returns to normal. You wonder why you were so worried and cancel the appointment (if you made one) until the next weird thing happens.

This is all perfectly fine (maybe not with you, but with Mother Nature) — it's all part of perimenopause.

Emotional emotions

For some women, it's not the disrupted sleep, hot flashes, or palpitations that get their attention — it's the mood swings. And thank goodness for loved ones who are right there to let us know just how irritable and unpleasant we've been. Welcome to perimenopause.

Mental miscues

You're already familiar with the roles hormones play in your mental agility and emotional stability because you've dealt with menstrual cycles and, in some cases, pregnancy. When estrogen levels drop and progesterone levels rise before your period, you get those annoying PMS symptoms such as fuzzy thinking, mood swings, fatigue, and restless sleep.

As hormone levels jump around during perimenopause, these annoying symptoms may become more commonplace. Estrogen has a role in managing a number of brain operations, and when estrogen levels take a dive during perimenopause, it's like guiding a boat that periodically loses its rudder. Here are some of the mental functions that estrogen helps manage (and some of the symptoms you may experience when estrogen takes a dive):

- Serotonin production. (*Serotonin* regulates sleep, pain, libido, mood, and other mental functions. Less estrogen can mean problems in all of these areas.)
- Body-temperature control. (You experience hot flashes and night sweats.)
- Pain threshold. (You're more sensitive or intolerant to pain.)
- Attention, mental focus, and concentration abilities. (You have mental lapses.)
- Communication between nerve cells related to memory. (You become forgetful.)

Meeting menopause

The onset of menopause, by definition, takes place a year after your last period. Very few medical conditions use an anniversary date as a basis for diagnosis, but lucky us, menopause is one. That's why figuring out who's in the club and who's not is so hard. After menopause, you're technically *postmenopausal* (for the rest of your life). The term *postmenopausal* hasn't really caught on in common usage (maybe because it's such a mouthful). So we generally use the term *menopause* to refer both to menopause and the postmenopausal years.

As far as your body is concerned, reaching menopause is almost a nonevent. Your ovaries have been slowing down for several years, producing lower and lower levels of estrogen and only releasing eggs sporadically.

Most of the symptoms ascribed to menopause generally begin during perimenopause. But back-to-back (to back) years of lower estrogen-production levels can result in health issues that you don't notice until menopause proper has set in. Over time, lower levels of estrogen (estradiol in particular) contribute to osteoporosis, cardiovascular problems, and other diseases. Due to these possible complications later in life, gynecologists and internists begin measuring your height, keeping a closer eye on your cholesterol levels and blood pressure readings, and monitoring your lifestyle habits (like exercise and diet) as you approach midlife.

Menopause is the time to review your diet, exercise routine, and unhealthy habits (smoking or excessive consumption of alcohol, for example). In your earlier life, your body was very forgiving. During menopause, it won't let you get away with unhealthy habits — you'll pay. During menopause, gaining weight is easier, and losing it is harder. And getting a good night's sleep and waking up feeling refreshed and ready to take on the day isn't as easy as it used to be. Make some healthy resolutions and stick with them so you don't wind up saying, like composer Eubie Blake said when he turned 100, "If I'd known I was going to live this long, I'd have taken better care of myself."

Prepping for Surgical Menopause

Surgical removal of your ovaries is a shock to your body. If you have both ovaries removed, you immediately go into menopause. This process is called *surgical menopause*. Instead of the gradual transition through perimenopause into menopause, you pop the clutch and go spinning into menopause. Your hormone levels drop instantaneously, except for those produced in the adrenal gland — testosterone and estrone.

To save you from a sudden, complete absence of hormones, your doctor will most likely give you hormones prior to surgery to allow your body to transition more smoothly to the new state of affairs. If you've had your ovaries removed, take note: Some experts believe that you're at greater risk of osteoporosis and heart disease. (Check out Chapters 4 and 5, respectively, for more on these conditions.)

Women who have only one ovary removed may go through a normal, natural menopause if the other ovary works properly. One ovary can produce eggs for a pregnancy and hormones to keep your body in good shape.

A *hysterectomy* (removal of your uterus) technically shouldn't slow down your ovaries' production of hormones. You should go through a natural menopause (though perhaps a little sooner) because your ovaries are still intact and producing hormones. Women with hysterectomies often go through menopause one to three years earlier than women without a hysterectomy.

We define menopause as reaching the one-year anniversary of your last period. But your uterus is gone, so you don't have a period. How do you know when you clear that hurdle? The only way to know is by watching the other symptoms — the restless-sleep habits, hot flashes, heart palpitations, and on, and on. If you experience the classic perimenopausal symptoms, you're probably entering perimenopause and your hormones are hopping up and sinking low. You're probably menopausal when your symptoms settle down.

Chapter 3

Getting in Sync with the Symptoms

You're irritable for no reason, you have trouble sleeping, you experience heart palpitations, and your sex drive is getting a little crazy. Sound familiar? If so, you're almost certainly starting down the road to menopause.

Every human body is unique — that's no surprise. But the path to menopause reveals just how different we really are. Some women breeze through the change, experiencing very few physical or emotional indications that anything is happening. Other women experience disturbing symptoms for an extended period of time. Fortunately, the symptoms often pass as you move into menopause and beyond.

In this chapter, we provide an introduction to the perimenopausal and menopausal symptoms you may experience. We go into much greater detail concerning the biology of menopause and how to alleviate these symptoms in other chapters of this book.

The symptoms we discuss in this chapter are all symptoms of perimenopause or menopause, but they're not unique to perimenopause and menopause. Other medical conditions cause these symptoms as well. If you experience any of these symptoms, don't just assume that they're a result of perimenopause or menopause. Your doctor will want to check out other possible causes.

Kicking Things Off with Perimenopausal Symptoms

In this section we give you the laundry list of symptoms that have been attributed to the sudden drops of estrogen during perimenopause. Women experience none, a few, or quite a few of these symptoms to greater or lesser degrees. If you think we sound wishy-washy, we're guilty as charged, but we have to hedge our bets because people are so very unique.

Those of you who have yet to experience perimenopause or menopause will take heart in the following statistic, but those of you who are currently experiencing symptoms may want to hide this statistic from the folks you live with — only 40 to 60 percent of women in the United States report experiencing any perimenopausal symptoms. For women who do experience symptoms, the symptoms can range in severity from being somewhat annoying to interfering with their ability to enjoy life.

Getting physical

When you heard Olivia Newton-John belt out "Let's get physical" a million years ago, did you ever think that it would come down to this? We surely didn't, but it has, so we need to outline the physical side of perimenopause — as in the outward, physical signs that your body's hormones are a-changing.

Many of the physical symptoms are the result of a string of events that happens when *estradiol* (the active form of estrogen) levels suddenly drop — a typical occurrence during perimenopause. The drop causes a chain reaction in your body, which we describe in the "Revealing the biology behind the symptoms" sidebar later in this chapter.

The relationship between estrogen and serotonin plays a role in many of the mental symptoms, but it also has a hand in some of the physical symptoms — like interrupted sleep. *Serotonin* is a compound that helps the body regulate sleep and moods. Though all the details aren't in, estrogen plays some kind of role in the production and maintenance of serotonin. It's amazing how all this stuff gets connected, huh?

Turning up the heat

Hot flashes (also called hot flushes) are the traditional, highly recognized symptom of menopause. When you have a hot flash, you suddenly feel very flushed — especially in your face and upper body. Increased perspiration usually accompanies this feeling of warmth. And, sometimes, dizziness, heart palpitations, and a suffocating feeling can precede or accompany hot flashes.

A sudden drop in estrogen levels triggers a hot flash. This drop in estrogen sends a message to your brain that something is terribly wrong, so your brain sends out a power burst of adrenaline (norepinephrine). *Norepinephrine* is the hormone that triggers the fight-or-flight response in humans, so your body moves into ready mode, which gets your blood pressure up and your heart pounding and also causes the blood vessels in your head, neck, and chest to dilate. All this commotion makes you feel like you're sweltering.

Until 1970, doctors didn't recognize hot flashes as a real physical phenomenon; they attributed the sensation to a woman's imagination or to a psychological problem.

Sweating your lack of sleep

Night sweats are essentially hot flashes that occur at night. The same estrogen drop that triggers hot flashes during the day triggers night sweats.

Night sweats can also be caused by infection, thyroid problems, or other types of illness, so if this is the only seemingly perimenopausal symptom you experience, check with your doctor.

Losing your snoozing time

With all the weird symptoms going on during the day, getting a good night's sleep so you can wake up feeling rested doesn't seem like a lot to ask for, but sometimes sleep can be a problem. Hot flashes in the middle of the night often result in interrupted sleep. You wake up, often perspiring (and sometimes cursing), and have a hard time going back to sleep. Interrupted sleep can cause sleep deprivation, which in turn leads to irritability, anxiety, and mood swings.

A rapid drop in estrogen also affects your serotonin levels. Serotonin helps regulate mood and sleep patterns. (Drugs such as Prozac and Zoloft work on the principle that serotonin regulation is key to relieving mood swings, irritability, and so on.) Estrogen makes serotonin more available by prolonging its action. When estrogen drops, it effects your serotonin levels, which contributes to interrupted sleep.

Getting to the heart of the palpitation issue

Butterflies in your stomach often accompany heart flutters, or *palpitations*. The sudden drops in estrogen that are so common during perimenopause cause reactions all over your body (see the "Revealing the biology behind the symptoms" sidebar later in this chapter), including heart flutters. The drop in estrogen causes your body's natural painkillers and mood regulators (*endorphins*) to drop. Your body interprets this state of affairs as trouble, so a command is issued to send out a burst of adrenaline (norepinephrine, the fight-or-flight hormone). Your body is responding as though you had just encountered a big grizzly bear. The only trouble is you don't see the grizzly bear, and you're left wondering why your body suddenly decided to get ready to flee from it just when you sat down to a nice candle-lit dinner.

Expecting menstrual irregularities

The approach to menopause can be blamed for a number of menstrual irregularities. But remember that you can't blame all irregularities on perimenopause. Although these menstrual symptoms often wait for women on the road to the change, consult your healthcare provider about these and all other symptoms before simply writing them off to perimenopause.

- ✔ **Irregular periods** are quite common in perimenopausal women because fluctuating hormone levels can interrupt the ovulation cycle. Some months you ovulate; some months you don't. If you don't ovulate, you don't produce enough progesterone to have a period, so the lining of your uterus builds up.

- ✔ **Heavy bleeding** during perimenopause is usually caused by an "eggless" cycle. You make estrogen during the first part of your cycle, but for some reason (often unknown), you just don't ovulate. Therefore, you don't produce progesterone, and you develop an unusually thick uterine lining, which you shed during your period. This process translates into abnormally heavy bleeding.

- ✔ **Bad timing** has probably struck every woman at one point or another. We just don't want you to think that perimenopause is going to make dealing with your periods easier. As long as you still have periods, they're liable to show up at inconvenient times. (A fact that makes getting rid of them not sound like a bad thing at all.)

Handling the headaches

For women who experience intense headaches during the first few days of their periods, we have some bad news — you may have more headaches during perimenopause. Headaches during the first few days of your period mean that you're sensitive to low estrogen levels, which are typical at that time. When estrogen levels drop quickly, which happens during perimenopause, the drop may trigger another one of those headaches.

Facing the fibroid factoids

Fibroids are simply balls of uterine muscle tissue. Nearly one-third of women have fibroids by the time they're 50. Fibroids tend to get bigger as you approach menopause, but they usually don't grow in size after menopause.

You really don't need to do anything about fibroids unless they cause symptoms such as pain, pressure, or increased bleeding.

Playing head games

The mental/emotional symptoms associated with perimenopause can be very frustrating given that many women don't associate their recent irritability or depression with perimenopause.

Revealing the biology behind the symptoms

As you may have suspected, the symptoms of menopause are all tied to plunging hormone levels. You may feel these symptoms more frequently during perimenopause than menopause because your hormone levels fluctuate more during perimenopause. Sometimes they rise to fairly normal levels, and then, they come crashing down. The *fluctuation* is the trigger for a lot of the symptoms. In menopause, hormone levels are consistently lower than they are during your reproductive years, so they don't pop up and drop down so frequently, though symptoms can still occur.

Here's a step-by-step guide of what happens to your body when your estradiol (the active form of estrogen) levels drop:

1. Your ovaries produce lower levels of estradiol, which causes a drop in the amount of estradiol reaching the brain.

2. Less estradiol in the brain causes a decrease in your endorphin levels. *Endorphins* are your body's natural painkillers and mood regulators. (If you're a runner, you're probably familiar with the effects of endorphins — they cause the "runner's high.")

3. Lower levels of endorphins in your brain cause it to think that something is terribly wrong, so it sends out a burst of adrenaline, namely *norepinephrine* (the hormone that triggers the fight-or-flight response).

4. The burst of norepinephrine causes your body to kick into ready-for-anything mode by increasing your heart rate (which causes those palpitations and flutters), raising your blood pressure, and dilating your blood vessels. Dilating blood vessels cause the hot flashes and sweating. If you're asleep, you may wake up suddenly. You may also experience diarrhea or get a feeling of anxiety and butterflies in your stomach.

The symptoms we list generally pass after your hormones settle into their new, lower levels after menopause. However, these symptoms severely inconvenience or otherwise bother many women during perimenopause. If this description mirrors your situation, there's no need sit there suffering in silence.

Be sure to inform your medical professional about these mental and emotional symptoms. They may be more closely related to hormonal imbalances than to psychological issues. But, either way, your healthcare professional can ensure that you get the proper treatment to alleviate your symptoms. (And, for more detailed information on the mental and emotional issues associated with perimenopause, check out Chapter 9.)

Sitting on the mood swings

Mood swings are common among perimenopausal women. But remember that mood swings are also common before your period (part of premenstrual syndrome) and after pregnancy. Although medical researchers don't know all the details, low levels of estrogen are associated with lower levels of serotonin, which can lead to mood swings, in addition to irritability, anxiety, pain sensitivity, eating disorders, and insomnia.

Worrying about anxiety

Anxiety is another common symptom perimenopausal women face. Like mood swings, anxiety seems to be tied to low levels of estrogen. The lower levels of endorphins and serotonin associated with low estrogen levels may trigger anxiety. Another theory is that low levels of estrogen, serotonin, and endorphins leave you more susceptible to the emotional stressors in your world. With this theory, lower estrogen, serotonin, and endorphin levels don't trigger anxiety; they simply inhibit your ability to easily deal with stressful situations.

Touching on irritability

The same hormonal shifts that cause mood swings and anxiety (see the previous "Sitting on the mood swings" and "Worrying about anxiety" sections) cause irritability. Like these other symptoms, irritability is a temporary condition that seems to blow over after you're menopausal (if you can put up with yourself for that long).

Recalling memory malfunctions

Memory problems during perimenopause sneak up on you. You forget your friend's name one day; you leave your keys somewhere in the grocery store another day. Pretty soon you start remembering how many times you couldn't remember something. We're not talking about dementia or Alzheimer's disease here; we're talking about forgetfulness and a lack of focus. This category covers relatively minor memory glitches: You forget where you're going with a thought in mid-sentence, or you get to the store and forget what you need to buy. Thank goodness for sticky notes and grocery lists.

Estrogen seems to facilitate communication among *neurons* (nerve cells) in the brain. Much of memory is a matter of the brain sending information from one memory storage center to another. Because estrogen helps maintain connections and grow new ones, shifting estrogen levels can stymie communication between memory storage areas. Memory problems seem to be a short-term issue; some women seem to lose the memory lapses after menopause.

We still don't know if hormones have anything to do with more permanent types of dementia or Alzheimer's disease. But the research is pointing in the direction that says estrogen could reduce the risk (or at least slow down the progression) of the Alzheimer's disease later in life.

Thinking through a haze

Fuzzy thinking is common when you're deprived of sleep or your hormones are in flux. When we say *fuzzy thinking,* we mean the feeling that you're just not with it today — like you're walking through a fog or you just can't concentrate on what you're doing. Fuzzy thinking can be the result of interrupted sleep (which isn't uncommon during perimenopause).

Fluctuating hormone levels also cause fuzzy thinking (as you may have experienced during pregnancy or at certain points in your menstrual cycle). Like many of the symptoms that accompany perimenopause, this too shall pass. Fuzzy thinking is a temporary thing. It generally clears up when your hormones settle down and your sleep patterns chill out during menopause.

Visiting the Menopausal Symptoms

All the symptoms we describe as *perimenopausal* have long been attributed to menopause. But after you're menopausal (without a menstrual period for a year), things begin to settle down a bit. Hot flashes subside and your moods stabilize. Your body and psyche seem to get used to some aspects of lower estrogen production.

The symptoms experienced after menopause are sometimes a bit more uncomfortable physically.

Long periods of low levels of estrogen encourage conditions such as osteoporosis, cardiovascular disease, heart attack, stroke, colon cancer, and other diseases discussed in Chapters 4 and 5 of this book.

To avoid wordiness, we use the term *menopause* in this chapter (and most others) to refer to the time period that incorporates both menopause and postmenopause.

Figuring out the physical facts

After your ovaries retire (well, they never really retire; they just greatly reduce their workload), you produce lower levels of estrogen without the sudden spikes and drops typical of perimenopause. Your hormones calm down — way down. As time goes by, these long periods of low estrogen levels result in some physical changes.

In this section, we discuss what these conditions feel like. We go into greater detail about the biology behind these conditions and how to alleviate the symptoms in other chapters of this book. (Chapter 6 deals with vaginal and urinary issues; Chapter 7 covers your skin and hair during menopause.)

Some of the symptoms are the result of lower levels of estrogen, pure and simple. We call these primary symptoms. Some of these primary symptoms can actually cause further unpleasantness, which we call secondary symptoms.

Peering into the primary symptoms

The primary symptoms include

- ✓ **Vaginal dryness:** The medical establishment refers to this condition as *vaginal atrophy.* Because estrogen keeps vaginal tissues moisturized and pliant, continuous periods of low estrogen can result in the drying out and shrinking of vaginal tissue. Between 20 and 45 percent of women in the United States experience vaginal dryness. They often notice it when intercourse becomes painful due to a lack of lubrication.

- ✓ **Vulvar discomfort:** Itching, burning, and dryness of the vulva isn't uncommon among menopausal women. But remember that many conditions and diseases that affect the vulva have nothing to do with estrogen, so have your doctor check out any vulvar changes.

- ✓ **Urinary incontinence:** This condition is much more prevalent in women after menopause than it is during the reproductive years. The tissues of your urinary tract become drier and thinner, and the muscles lose their tone as estrogen levels diminish. You know you're experiencing urinary incontinence if you have a hard time holding it when you laugh, exercise, or sneeze. Your urinary tract, especially your urethra, depends on estrogen to maintain its form and muscle tone. The urethra has a hard time sealing off the flow of urine after years of diminished estrogen levels.

- ✓ **Urinary frequency:** Like incontinence, urinary frequency results from sustained, low levels of estrogen that define menopause. Urinary frequency simply means that you have to urinate frequently. You may leave the bathroom and quickly feel like you have to go again. This condition can be very frustrating during the day — and even more frustrating at night. Urinary frequency can also cause interrupted sleep, which understandably, turns into irritability.

- ✓ **Skin changes:** Lower estrogen levels cause your skin to sag and wrinkle. Estrogen doesn't literally prevent sagging. But estrogen does keep your skin elastic and help your skin retain fluid, so it remains "filled out" rather than becoming loose and droopy.

- ✓ **Hair changes:** Your hair becomes thinner and more brittle with menopause, though some women report that their hair feels as soft and fluffy as cotton several years into menopause. Estrogen seems to be a natural moisturizer, so with lower levels of the stuff flowing through your body, your hair takes a hit and becomes more brittle. You also have a tougher time keeping a perm permanent.

- ✓ **Weight changes:** Your weight shifts to the center of your body — around your waist. Instead of the lovely pear-shaped body you once had, you take on more of an apple-shaped appearance due to shifting hormone levels. Although you may gain a bit of weight, you probably can't directly blame that on hormonal changes. Your body simply becomes less forgiving about nutritional imbalances and poor eating, drinking, and exercise habits.

Sniffing out the secondary conditions

It's not over yet. One or more of the primary symptoms can trigger even more unpleasantness. Here you go:

- **Painful intercourse:** Experiencing pain during intercourse is generally the result of vaginal dryness or physical changes in the position of the urethra due to changes in the shape of the vagina that happen over time when estrogen levels are continuously low. As low levels of estrogen cause your *urovaginal tissues* (tissues of the vagina and urinary tract) to become thinner and the supporting muscle to lose its tone, your organs naturally shift position a bit.

- **Interrupted sleep:** Hot flashes, urinary frequency, anxiety, and a variety of other menopausal symptoms can cause interrupted sleep during the night. You wake up feeling tired and experience fatigue throughout the day because your body isn't able to enter the deep stages of sleep at night.

- **Fatigue:** If you consistently don't get a good restful night's sleep or you experience insomnia, you may become fatigued. But fatigue can also be the result of low testosterone levels.

Discovering that it's more than skin deep

The mental/emotional aspects of menopause are more of a mixed bag. Some symptoms experienced during menopause usually decrease or go away completely; others are a bit more difficult to deal with.

- **Anxiety:** Often, the anxiety common during perimenopause is caused by the rapid drop in estrogen, which initiates a chain reaction (see the "Revealing the biology behind the symptoms" sidebar in this chapter). After menopause, unexplained anxiety often dies down, and you return to your normal self.

- **Depression:** Women who have had hysterectomies are more likely to experience menopause-related depression than women who go through a natural menopause. Researchers don't yet understand why this is the case.

  Also, women who have been on estrogen and suddenly quit taking it, rather than going through a weaning process, also have more problems with depression. Estrogen assists in the production of serotonin (a substance which helps regulate moods), so lower levels of estrogen can mean lower levels of serotonin.

- **Headaches:** Women who experience their first migraine during perimenopause often find that the migraines go away after menopause.

- **Lower libido:** Decreased sex drive is a problem for many menopausal women, but the good news is that 70 percent of women remain sexually active during their perimenopausal and menopausal years. Lower libido can be traced to hormonal imbalances and may be the result of testosterone levels being too low. (For more information on menopause and your libido, take a look at Chapter 8.)

✔ **Memory lapses and fuzzy thinking:** Though memory lapses and fuzzy thinking are common during perimenopause, most women notice their concentration and memory return to normal after menopause. Aging can cause mental impairment later in life, but you can't blame everything on menopause!

Unraveling the Mystery

Many people associate the word *symptom* with disease, but the definition we use throughout this book is much closer to the dictionary definition — a condition or event that accompanies something. Sometimes you only see perimenopause in your rear-view mirror. You may not know that you experienced perimenopause until years later.

But for many women, perimenopausal symptoms surface at one time or another. If you're like many women, you may feel that weird things keep happening to your body or your emotions. But it may take a little investigation on your part to bring the whole perimenopausal picture into focus.

Maybe you feel a flutter in your chest, and you become convinced that you're on the verge of a heart attack. If you go to a cardiologist to check out heart palpitations, she probably won't even think to check your hormones because she's looking for something in your heart to answer the riddle.

Or maybe the "weird things" going on with you aren't physical at all. Maybe they're emotional — like becoming easily frustrated at work or chewing your kids out 50 times a day for the last two weeks. Many women may think twice about these symptoms, but they don't bring them up with their doctor. If you do mention them to your doctor, she may say something like, "It's nothing." Nothing? We know what you're thinking, "Try telling that to my coworkers and my kids."

After you get a hot flash or two, you may figure out that these "weird things" aren't part of your imagination and that you're getting close to menopause. If you figure out the connection, consider yourself lucky. Few women realize that the heart palpitations and the irritability can be part of the same condition — perimenopause. Having read this book, you can be the local expert — it's up to you to coach other women through this!

Even gynecologists sometimes overlook a hormonal imbalance as the source of symptoms. Women may suspect that their problem is "chemical" or hormonal only to have doctors say that they're too young for menopause or that they're still having periods, so they aren't menopausal.

Some gynecologists go so far as to take a blood test to check your FSH (follicle stimulating hormone) level to rule out menopause. High levels of FSH are indicative of *menopause*. But during perimenopause, your hormone levels go up and down. One month your FSH may be perfectly normal; another month it may be high. Without getting tested month after month, determining whether you're *perimenopausal* is difficult.

But women's estrogen and testosterone levels can (and usually do) get out of whack even before they officially become menopausal, and the imbalance triggers the annoying symptoms often associated with menopause. Sometimes you can become even more frustrated after seeking medical advice because the experts tell you, "It's nothing," or they alarm you with the number and types of tests they want you to take.

The reality is that the symptoms you experience are often more intense before menopause, during perimenopause, than they are after you make the change.

Part II

The Effects of Menopause on Your Body and Mind

The 5th Wave   By Rich Tennant

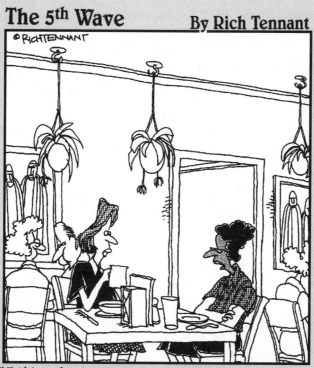

"I think they're typical symptoms of menopause – gaining weight, feeling tired, locking your husband in the basement because he finished the double-chunk peanut butter."

In this part . . .

Are you convinced that the goldfish is deliberately trying to aggravate you? Has your family recently taken to wearing gloves and parkas in the house in August because you insist on keeping the air-conditioning cranked all the way up? We jest because we've been there. But the years before and after menopause can bring a whole host of symptoms and conditions with them — from the simply annoying to the potentially dangerous. Don't worry: Knowledge is power! In this part, we cover the physical, mental, and emotional symptoms and conditions that women run into. We deal with your bones, cardiovascular system, female organs, skin, hair, sex life, and mental and emotional outlook. Pretty thorough, huh?

Chapter 4

The Business of Your Bones

In This Chapter

▶ Understanding how bone stays healthy

▶ Recognizing estrogen's role in bone loss

▶ Understanding the medical tests that help identify osteoporosis

▶ Discovering why women are at greater risk of developing osteoporosis after menopause

Most of us don't want to just live through menopause, we want to dance through it and keep dancing for another 40 or 50 years. Healthy bones keep your get-up-and-go from turning into sit-down-and-wait.

Osteoporosis literally means "porous bone." It's a disease in which your bones become thin and fragile and more likely to break. In fact, bones can become so fragile that they're crushed by their own weight. When the grocery clerk throws apples on top of the soft bread in your grocery bag, the bread becomes smashed and deformed from the weight of the apples. A similar thing happens when your bones in your back press on each other — you develop a hump.

You can lower your risk of developing osteoporosis by building healthy bones before menopause and making some healthy choices in your lifestyle after menopause.

Why are women more susceptible to osteoporosis after menopause? Why are women more prone to osteoporosis than men? What's the connection between estrogen and osteoporosis? What can you do after menopause to save your bones? You can discover the answers to these questions in this chapter and find ways to keep your bones dancing through menopause.

Homing In on Bone Health

Knowing how your body makes bones and what it takes to keep them healthy is a good place to start when outlining the relationship between the change and the health of your bones. Your bones don't quit growing after you become an adult. They're alive and changing throughout your life.

Growing big bones and strong bones

When you're a kid, it's obvious that your bones are growing. As your bones get longer, you get taller. But your bones don't just grow longer; they also get thicker — denser. The denser the bone, the harder it is to break. Think of your dinnerware. Those thick earthenware plates are much more difficult to break than the fragile, translucent, fine china found in expensive restaurants. People with strong bones have dense bones. Your bones continue to increase in density until you're about 30 years old, at which age you reach *peak bone density.* The goal of all young women should be to try to make their bones more like earthenware than fine china by the time they reach 30. If you start building strong, dense bones when you're young, the effects of bone loss in midlife are less problematic. The higher your peak bone density, the better chance you have of keeping your bones healthy.

In the animal kingdom, males tend to be bigger than females; men also tend to have denser bones than women. On average, African-American women have denser bones than Caucasian and Asian women. This is why men and African-American women generally have less trouble with osteoporosis than Caucasian and Asian women.

TECHNICAL STUFF

Remodeling your house of bones

To better understand osteoporosis, it helps to look at how bone is "built." Each bone contains cells that build bone (*osteoblasts*) and cells that clear away bone (*osteoclasts*). This setup may sound familiar if you've ever undertaken a home-remodeling project. One crew comes in to knock down walls, and then (a month after the first crew trashed your house), another crew comes in to build the new room. Even medical professionals refer to the bone-growing process as "remodeling" because it serves the same purpose as remodeling a house. This life-long, bone-remodeling process helps maintain healthy bone by fixing wear and tear caused by everyday living.

At some point, a section of bone is selected as a remodeling site. (Scientists don't know much about how the site gets selected.) Osteoclasts remove bone by dissolving it with acid, which creates a cavity. This process of breaking down

bone is referred to as bone *resorption.* What happens to the dissolved bone? The body is an efficient recycler — the calcium and other minerals that made up the bone pass into the blood-stream and are used by other parts of the body. In fact, whenever your body needs extra calcium, the osteoclasts get busy dissolving more bone. That's why it's important to keep the body well supplied with calcium so your osteoclasts don't cannibalize your bones for calcium.

After the osteoclasts have done their thing, the osteoblasts get to work building new bone by spreading a gel-like substance in the cavity. Over the course of a month, this gel hardens into bone. The bone-remodeling project takes about two to three months. That's probably quicker than your last home-remodeling project, but it's a slower healing process than those associated with other tissues such as muscle or skin.

Understanding peak bone density

Peak bone density is the maximum amount of bone that you'll ever have. Most people reach their peak by about age 30. Maximizing your peak bone density is important because, after 35, you lose more bone than you build.

Your peak bone density depends on a number of factors such as genetics, diet, and exercise. You can't control your genes — you're born with them. Among other things, genes control the size of your frame and your ability to produce bone. But you can control your diet to get plenty of calcium, vitamin D, and magnesium, and you can exercise early in life so that you maximize your peak bone density. Avoiding alcohol and smoking early in life also helps you reach a high peak bone density.

Keeping Pace with Bone Reconstruction

Even after you grow to your full height, your bones keep gaining and losing bone material. Your body's maintenance process, called *remodeling,* keeps your bones strong and healthy day in and day out. Hormones help regulate the maintenance process. So you can imagine that as your hormones change, it messes up the bone maintenance process. (Check out the "Remodeling your house of bones" sidebar in this chapter for the ins and outs of bone remodeling.)

During your first 30 years on this planet, bone building exceeds bone destruction in the remodeling process, and your bones stay nice and healthy. After the big 3-0 or thereabouts, the teardown crew stays active, but the builders have a harder time keeping up.

The builders don't quite fill in all the cavities created by the tear down crew, and the maintenance process becomes unbalanced. Like a washing machine with all the clothes clumped on one side, the cycle begins to break down. As the respective crews destroy more bone than they repair, your bones weaken, becoming less dense.

Making the calcium connection

Calcium is the central figure in the bone story. Your body needs calcium to build bones and to keep every cell in your body in shape. Calcium helps muscles contract, nerves respond, and blood clot. Bones store the calcium your body uses until they release the calcium to a part of the body that requests it.

Table 4-1 lists calcium requirements by age. As your bones grow larger, your body needs more calcium. Your calcium requirements level off during your reproductive years but increase after menopause. The reason — estrogen helps your body absorb the calcium in your food. What happens to the calcium that's not absorbed? It goes out with the trash (other waste products). So to get the same amount of calcium into your bones, you have to take in more calcium.

Table 4-1	Calcium Requirements by Age
Age	*Calcium Recommendation (in Milligrams)*
1–3	500
4–8	800
9–18	1,300
19–50	1,000
51 and older	1,200

When you eat a food or a food supplement rich in calcium, the calcium doesn't automatically go to your bones. It must be digested and absorbed by your body to help your bones and other tissues that need it.

You may think that keeping your bones building and rebuilding is simply a matter of getting enough calcium, and you'd be partly right, but a number of vitamins and hormones help your body digest and absorb calcium. These vitamins and hormones have to be working right for the calcium in your diet to get incorporated into your bones (see the "Nutrition" section later in this chapter).

If the calcium in your blood drops below a certain level, your *parathyroid glands,* which monitor the amount of calcium in your blood, send the parathyroid hormone out into the bloodstream to deliver messages to your kidneys and your osteoclasts.

✔ Your kidneys get a message: "Save the calcium, don't put it in the urine!" In response, your helpful kidneys start activating the vitamin D they've been storing so you can better absorb the calcium you eat.

✔ Your *osteoclasts* (the destruction crew) get a message: "Start mining calcium from the bones to beef up supplies in the bloodstream."

Your body cannibalizes its own bone to supply calcium to other cells if it doesn't get enough calcium or vitamin D. As a result, you suffer bone loss.

There are two ways to skin this cat: Either get more calcium in your diet or slow down the remodeling process so that the builders can keep up with the

Attention pregnant and nursing moms

Your body demands even more calcium than normal during pregnancy and while you're breast-feeding. Although hormonal changes during pregnancy help your body absorb calcium more efficiently, if you're not getting enough calcium, your body makes up for it by dissolving bone. If you have a multiple pregnancy or closely spaced pregnancies, be sure you get enough calcium and vitamin D. Getting sufficient quantities of these nutrients usually requires taking food supplements in addition to pregnancy vitamins.

Breast-feeding, particularly if you breast-feed for more than six months, also depletes your body of calcium. You have two concerns in this situation:

✔ You want to make sure that your milk contains enough calcium to properly nourish your baby.

✔ You want to make sure that the calcium supply comes from your diet, not your bones.

Fortunately, nature takes care of the first concern. Unfortunately, your bones may suffer as a result. If you don't have sufficient calcium for your baby, your body pulls calcium from your bones. Although they're controversial, some studies show that moms can lose up to 5 percent of their bone mass while breast-feeding. Again, calcium and vitamin D supplements in addition to pregnancy vitamins are critical.

destruction crew. You can get more calcium into your system by taking supplements and exercising. To slow down the destruction crew, you need medication (see the "Treating Osteoporosis" section later on).

Recognizing the role of sex hormones

Your body needs vitamins to absorb calcium, but sex hormones also play a big role in helping your body absorb the calcium you eat and manage the remodeling process. Because your body produces less estrogen after the change, your hormones are thrown out of the balance. The imbalance affects your bones.

Estrogen helps absorb the calcium and magnesium you eat and deposits it properly into your skeleton to give you strong bones. Estrogen also has a calming effect on bone destruction and lets the bone builders catch up with the bone destroyers. As your estrogen supply dwindles during menopause, the bone destroyers get more active. What's more, you aren't able to digest as much of the calcium and magnesium you get from your food as your estrogen supply declines. If you continue eating like you have in the past, the same amount of calcium and magnesium won't go nearly as far in helping to build bone. That's why most women add calcium and magnesium supplements to their diet after menopause.

Some of the other sex hormones that help in the bone building process include progesterone and testosterone, both of which your ovaries produce.

Latest research on estrogen and osteoporosis

Cytokines may help us figure out how estrogen slows down the bone destruction that leads to osteoporosis. *Cytokines* are substances inside the bone that regulate immune response. Some of the latest research shows that they may also regulate the osteoblasts and osteoclasts, the bone builders and destroyers.

So far, researchers know that one of these cytokines, *interleukin-6,* rises after menopause. They also know that the teardown crew (osteoclasts) becomes even more active after menopause if a woman doesn't take hormone therapy (HT). Putting two and two together, it may be that a rise in interleukin-6 causes the osteoclasts to more actively destroy bone. Estrogen replacement reduces interleukin-6, and it also stops bone loss. Is this a coincidence? Scientists are trying to determine if there's a connection and if other interleukins are involved.

✔ Testosterone is actually a better bone builder than progesterone. It not only triggers the osteoblasts to build bone, but it also helps them build stronger bones.

✔ Progesterone helps the bone builders repair bone, but only if estrogen is present.

The slowdown of estrogen and testosterone production is another one of the reasons the bone builders have a hard time keeping up with the destruction crew after menopause.

So, sex hormones are an important player in the osteoporosis game because they regulate bone remodeling. If you let the bone destroyers get too rowdy and don't force the bone builders to keep up with them, bone deteriorates and becomes less dense.

Boning Up on Osteoporosis

Osteoporosis is a disease characterized by weak and brittle bones. Bone deteriorates, as you grow older, becoming weak and brittle. Anyone lucky enough to live to a ripe, old age loses bone — it's part of the natural aging process. But not everyone develops osteoporosis. Osteoporosis is a serious issue for women — particularly during and after menopause.

The real danger of osteoporosis is that it sets the stage for literally breaking a leg (or a hip, or a wrist, or another bone). And as you age, breaking a bone becomes more than an inconvenience — it can be deadly. A hip fracture carries the same mortality rate as breast cancer in the elderly! And half of hip-fracture victims become dependent upon caregivers for the rest of their lives.

Linking osteoporosis and women

There's good news and bad news about osteoporosis and women. We're going to get the bad news out of the way first: About 25 million Americans have osteoporosis, and most of them are women. The good news is that the disease is preventable and treatable, even after menopause.

Women lose bone at very different rates, so the following generalizations reflect averages for the *perimenopausal* (premenopausal), menopausal, and postmenopausal years and don't necessarily apply to every woman:

- **Perimenopause:** Most women begin losing bone from their spine before or during perimenopause at a rate of 1 percent per year.

- **Menopause:** After a woman becomes menopausal, the rate of bone loss increases to about 3 percent per year if she doesn't receive hormone therapy.

- **Postmenopause:** Sometime during the ten years following menopause, bone loss slows back down to a rate of about 1 percent per year.

In the first five to seven years following menopause, a woman can lose as much as 20 percent of the total bone she's expected to lose during her life-time. By the time a woman is in her eighties, she may have lost as much as 47 percent of her total bone density.

After reading all that, you can probably use some good news. Well, here it is: Only 25 to 33 percent of women develop osteoporosis. However, it's like a thunderstorm. You may only have a 33 percent chance of rain, but if it rains on your picnic, it's a mess.

Defining and diagnosing osteoporosis

Osteoporosis literally means porous bone — bone that is weak and brittle. Too little calcium in the bone is the cause of this disease. Both men and women can develop osteoporosis, but it's more common in women than men for a couple of reasons:

- ✔ Women's bones are less dense than men's bones.

- ✔ Testosterone stimulates bone growth and helps build stronger bones. Men have more testosterone than women.

- ✔ More women live further into their senior years than men.

In your grandmother's day, doctors only diagnosed patients as having osteoporosis if they actually broke a bone because of the disease. Waiting for a fracture before taking action is like buying a lottery ticket after the drawing — it's a bit too late. Today, technology exists that can help identify osteoporosis before it results in painful and often debilitating fractures.

Diagnosing osteoporosis in terms of objective measurements of bone density is more practical than waiting for an injury. Bone-density measurements allow your medical team to treat your condition early so you can prevent injury and promote healing. We baby boomers are definitely into prevention.

How can you tell a healthy bone from a fragile bone? One way is to cut the bone in half and look at a cross-section (as we illustrate in Figure 4-1).

- ✔ A healthy bone looks like Swiss cheese — lots of cheese separated by small holes.

- ✔ A fragile bone looks like lace — lots of holes separated by thin, string-like structures.

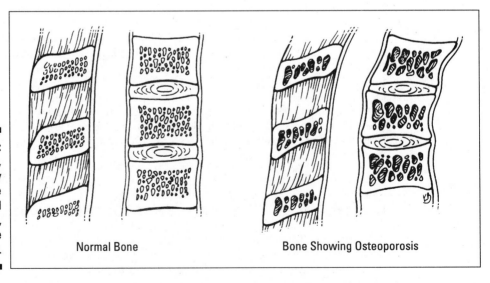

Figure 4-1: Normal, cheesy bone on the left and breakable, lacy bone on the right.

Normal Bone   Bone Showing Osteoporosis

Medical folks measure bone density (strength) to determine if you have brittle bones. Nearly 30 years of research has proven that low bone density leads to fractures.

Osteoporosis today is defined in terms of how your bone density compares with the peak bone density of a healthy, 35-year-old woman, which serves as the basis for the Young Adult category in Table 4-2.

✓ If your bones are just slightly less dense than the bones of an average 35-year-old, the diagnosis is *osteopenia* — low bone density.

✓ If they're significantly less dense than the bones of an average 35-year-old, the diagnosis is *osteoporosis* — brittle bones. Table 4-2 shows the National Osteoporosis Foundation's criteria used to diagnose osteoporosis as of 1998.

Table 4-2	Criteria for Diagnosing Osteoporosis
Category	*Bone Density T-Score*
Normal	Less than 1.0 standard deviation below Young Adult
Osteopenia	1.0–2.5 standard deviations below Young Adult
Osteoporosis	2.5 or more standard deviations below Young Adult
Severe osteoporosis	2.0 or more standard deviations below Young Adult and evidence of fractures

The threshold that separates osteopenia from full-blown osteoporosis comes from research that shows how much bone you can lose before significantly increasing your risk of fracture. Folks with osteoporosis have low bone density, but they also have a higher risk of fracturing a bone.

Looking at causes

Sixty years ago, doctors noticed that osteoporosis occurred primarily in menopausal women. They suspected that osteoporosis was related to sex hormones — specifically a deficiency of estrogen. Hundreds of research grants later, medical professionals and ordinary folks know that estrogen levels affect bone density.

Does menopause *cause* osteoporosis? The short answer is no. Osteoporosis is caused by calcium deficiency in the bones, and estrogen plays a role in getting calcium to your bones and keeping bones healthy. (Check out the "Making the calcium connection" section earlier in this chapter for more on calcium's role.)

Deficiencies of other vitamins, minerals, and hormones can influence the amount of calcium that gets absorbed by your bone, thereby contributing to the development of osteoporosis. Lack of exercise can promote osteoporosis as well. Finally, lifestyle choices, such as the use of tobacco and alcohol, can also play a role in the onset of osteoporosis.

Avoiding the effects

Osteoporosis weakens every bone in your body, leaving them prone to breaking. The bones most likely to break include the spine, hip, and wrist bones. Breaking your wrist may inconvenience you for a few weeks or months. Hip fractures are much more debilitating. Crushed vertebrae, so often associated with osteoporosis, can cause you to become shorter. Crushed vertebrae can leave you with a stooped appearance too.

✔ **Spinal fractures:** Fractures of the spine aren't technically breaks; they're compressions. The weight of your body crushes, or compresses, the round body of the vertebra, which provides these fractures with their name, *compression fractures.* Compression fractures in your spine can leave you stooped with what appears to be a hump in your back (called a *dowager's hump*).

Between 5 and 15 percent of 50-year-old women get compression fractures in their spine. By age 70, that number grows to between 40 and 55 percent. (It depends on whose research you're looking at.) Often, these crushed or wedged vertebrae cause little or no pain. You simply begin to notice poor posture that you can't corrected by standing up as straight as you can.

You may notice the first sign of crushed vertebrae during your annual medical exam. After the age of 40 or 45 your doctor starts measuring your height. Women with crushed or wedged vertebrae are often shorter than they were before. If you find yourself getting shorter, the measurement may not be a mistake — it could be a sign of osteoporosis. Figure 4-2 shows the possible changes in your spine that accompany osteoporosis.

Although most women experience little or no pain when the vertebrae collapse, some women do. You can usually control the pain by using an over-the-counter painkiller like ibuprofen or aspirin. The pain rarely lasts more than a few months.

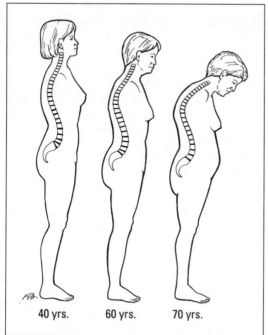

Figure 4-2:
The
shrinking
effects of
osteo-
porosis.

40 yrs.   60 yrs.   70 yrs.

✔ **Hip fractures:** This problem is generally the result of a fall that breaks the *femur,* the long bone of the thigh that connects your knee to your hip. This break often occurs at the head of the femur where it connects to the hip socket.

More than 90 percent of hip fractures occur in people over 70. So even though osteoporosis can begin during perimenopause, it can be corrected or held at bay so that you don't experience the debilitating aspects of the disease — the fractures. But don't underestimate the trauma of experiencing a broken hip at age 70. Only one-third of all women who have hip fractures regain the functionality they had prior to the fracture. Another third wind up in nursing homes. And unfortunately, about 20 percent die of complications within a year of the fracture.

✔ **Wrist fractures:** Wrist fractures are common. When you fall, your first reaction is to catch yourself by sticking your hands out in front of you. You don't have to guess why wrist fractures are common in women with osteoporosis.

Preventing Osteoporosis by Managing Your Risk Factors

Your risk of developing osteoporosis is higher than your risk of getting breast, ovarian, or uterine cancer combined. After your 50th birthday, your risk of developing osteoporosis grows. One out of two Caucasian women over 50 will sustain a fracture due to osteoporosis in her lifetime. That's nearly twice as high as the fracture rate for African-American women. So, the next time you're sitting in a Mother's Club meeting, look to one side. Depending on your ethnicity, it's likely that either you or the friend next to you will break a bone because of osteoporosis.

Some women develop osteoporosis as they age, and others don't. It's important to understand why this happens and how to be one of the women who doesn't fall victim to this disease.

If you're a young woman, you can start preventing osteoporosis today. If you're over 35, finding out how healthy your bones are right now is a good place to start. In either case, prevention and treatment are easier if you understand how your bones stay healthy, how osteoporosis develops, and why your risk of developing brittle bones increases after menopause. (Check out the preceding "Keeping Pace with Bone Reconstruction" section.)

Risk factors vary by age. From childhood through your twenties, you can lower your risk of osteoporosis by getting enough calcium, vitamins, and minerals; by exercising; and by avoiding unhealthy activities such as smoking and drinking alcohol. (We discuss exercise in Chapters 19 and 22.)

If you have children (whether they're toddlers or young adults), they can begin taking measures right away to prevent this disease. The stronger your bones are early in life, the more you have to work with as you grow older. Having really dense bones when your bone density peaks (when you're about 30) gives you more bone to work with during and after menopause. Young people can develop strong bones by eating properly and staying fit (see Chapters 18 and 19).

After your thirties are in your rearview mirror and you begin to go through perimenopause and menopause, menopausal-related shifts in sex hormones and other factors increase your risk of osteoporosis. (Check out the "Recognizing the role of sex hormones" section earlier in this chapter for more on the connection between osteoporosis and these hormones.) Risk factors boil down to three basic categories:

> ✔ Genetic factors and family background
>
> ✔ Personal health history
>
> ✔ Your lifestyle

We devote a subsection to each of these topics.

Blaming your genes: Genetic factors and family background

Your genes establish a lot of the rules concerning how your body develops and how it ages. So it's no surprise that genetics plays a role in increasing or reducing your risk of osteoporosis.

Caucasian and Asian women have higher risks of osteoporosis than women of African ancestry, particularly during perimenopause and the early years of menopause. African Americans have a 6 percent lifetime risk of osteoporosis, but Caucasian and Asian women each have a lifetime risk of about 14 percent. The lower incidence of osteoporosis in African-American women is probably due to the fact that African-American women have higher peak bone densities than Caucasian and Asian women. Even though everyone loses bone with age, African-American women have the advantage of having stronger bones from the start.

Body build

Large-boned people generally build more bone than small-framed people, and they often start out with more bone mass when they hit their bone-building peak. As they age, large-boned people draw from a larger supply of calcium, so bone deterioration takes longer. But large-boned people aren't completely safe; they get osteoporosis too. Small-boned, or petite, women have lower peak bone densities, so they have less bone to lose.

Family history of osteoporosis

Medical folks have found that daughters of osteoporosis sufferers tend to have lower peak bone density than normal for their age. Because of their genes, some women just don't make as much bone even with a proper diet and exercise. Genes help determine our ability to make bone.

Reviewing your personal health history

A number of aspects of your personal history influence your risk of osteoporosis, including menstrual and menopause-related issues and the medications that you take.

Menstruation

Because estrogen prevents bone loss, the more estrogen you produce during your lifetime, the less your risk of osteoporosis. Not surprisingly, many factors relating to your periods affect how much estrogen you produce and, therefore, your risk for osteoporosis. Check out the following:

- ✔ **Age at your first period:** After you begin menstruation, your body produces more estrogen. Most girls begin to menstruate sometime between the ages of 11½ and 13. If you get your period early, you may produce more estrogen in your lifetime than the average woman. With the additional estrogen, your bones may have a higher peak bone density than the average woman. Of course, this assumes that you followed a proper diet and got appropriate amounts of exercise. If you start out with higher bone density, you can lower your risk for osteoporosis.

- ✔ **Age at the onset of menopause:** Most women go through menopause between the ages of 45 and 55. Women who go through menopause earlier, whether naturally or because of surgery, begin losing bone earlier than women who start the change later in life. You produce lower levels of estrogen earlier, so your risk of osteoporosis goes up.

    Your body produces much less estrogen after menopause than it did during your reproductive years, and the more estrogen you produce in your lifetime, the lower your risk of osteoporosis.

- ✔ **Ovary removal:** Women who have their ovaries removed (an *oophorectomy*) go through *surgical menopause,* which is exactly what it sounds like — immediate menopause caused by surgery. This sudden change jolts your system because you lose most of your hormones immediately and permanently. Women who have their ovaries removed have twice as much bone loss and a higher risk of osteoporosis than women with their ovaries. Women who have their ovaries removed before age 35 often develop osteoporosis even with hormone therapy.

- ✔ **Hysterectomy:** Women who have their uterus removed (*hysterectomy*) can go through menopause two years earlier than other women. The earlier onset probably results from cutting off some of the blood flow to the ovaries. The earlier onset of menopause increases your risk of osteoporosis a bit because you have fewer years of estrogen production.

Eating disorders

Anorexia and bulimia (along with over-exercising) can lead to low estrogen levels, which can cause you to skip periods and your body to begin losing more bone than it builds. Losing more bone than your body builds leads to osteoporosis.

Medications

Some medications affect peak bone density, raising your risk of osteoporosis. Ask your physician or read the literature that accompanies the medications to determine if you're at risk of bone loss from using a specific medication. Some of the medications that can affect your bones include

✔ Corticosteriods used to treat chronic conditions such as asthma, rheumatoid arthritis, and psoriasis can cause bone loss. These drugs increase bone loss by inhibiting calcium absorption. Women who take corticosteroid dosages greater than 5 milligrams for more than two months increase their risk of bone loss. Sometimes, physicians prescribe Fosamax, a drug that slows down bone destruction and encourages bone building, along with certain steroids if long-term steroid use is necessary.

✔ Too high a dosage of thyroid-replacement medication or an overactive thyroid (as with Grave's disease) can decrease bone strength. Excess thyroid hormone causes bone loss.

✔ Certain types of diuretics used to treat heart disease or high blood pressure cause the body to excrete more calcium. When used for prolonged periods of time, they can raise your risk of bone loss.

Thiazide diuretics, on the other hand, actually reduce the amount of calcium excreted in the urine. They also seem to inhibit bone breakdown.

Surgeries

Certain surgeries can increase your risk of osteoporosis because they impact your body's ability to absorb or digest calcium or the vitamins and minerals needed to get calcium from your diet into the bone. These surgeries include

✔ **Gastrectomy:** Removal of all or part of the stomach. This surgery impacts your ability to digest calcium and other nutrients needed to build bone.

✔ **Intestinal bypass:** Surgery to remove a portion of your intestine. This surgery impacts your ability to absorb calcium and other nutrients needed to build bone.

✔ **Thyroidectomy:** Surgery to remove part or all of the thyroid gland. If your thyroid is removed, you must take thyroid-hormone medication. Too much thyroid-replacement medication triggers excessive bone loss and a decrease in bone strength.

Looking to your lifestyle

Now we come to the section about lifestyle issues, most of which you have some control over. You can't do much about your age (even if you claim to be

39 years old for the rest of your life, your body knows the truth). But you can take steps to lower your risk of osteoporosis by picking up some new healthy habits and eliminating the unhealthy habits.

Age

From the time you're born until you're about 30, your main job is to build the strongest skeleton you can by following a healthful diet, exercising regularly, and avoiding tobacco and alcohol. After you reach your thirties, your body loses bone faster than it makes it.

By the time you're 70, you've probably lost about as much bone as you're going to, but other aspects of aging increase your risk of falling and breaking a bone. By 70 or 80, your body has lost much of its flexibility, you may have less balance, your eyesight and depth perception may be poor, and you may be taking medications that affect bone loss or physical conditioning.

Smoking

Smoking and using other tobacco products is unhealthy in every respect — not only because it decreases bone density. Tobacco use is especially unhealthy for children and adolescents. When children and adolescents smoke, they build less bone mass during a major developmental period in their lives. Because the use of tobacco decreases bone density, it's not a healthy habit during and after menopause either.

Alcohol use

More than three drinks a day is considered excessive as far as raising your risk of osteoporosis. Excessive alcohol consumption decreases bone density.

Exercise

Exercise is the kindest gift you can give your bones after you give them calcium. It's critical to building strong bones. Exercise puts stress on your bones, which is a good thing as far as bone density is concerned. Stress forces the bone tissue to absorb calcium; therefore, it gets stronger. Exercise also stimulates the muscles around the bone so that the muscles get stronger and put even more pressure on your bones.

The space program in the United States points to the importance of exercise in maintaining healthy bones. Scientists are very concerned with the effects of prolonged weightlessness on the astronauts' bones, so astronauts make sure to exercise while in orbit.

Exercise during childhood and early adulthood is important in preventing osteoporosis because it helps your bones achieve their full potential strength. Later in life, exercise helps your bones to continue to absorb calcium so that they stay strong.

Lack of exercise not only decreases bone density, it also makes you more susceptible to fractures. Women who exercise lower their risk of fracture by 30 percent.

Although physical activity helps protect your body against osteoporosis, too much strenuous activity can lead to low levels of estrogen. Unless you're training for the Olympics, you probably aren't exercising too strenuously. Skipping periods can be a sign that you're over-exercising.

Nutrition

Calcium helps your body build bone. But calcium does much more than the TV advertisements proclaim. Calcium is also fundamental to regulating your sleep and moods and to proper muscle function.

Dairy products are the best source of calcium as far as food goes. A variety of vegetables also contain calcium, but vegetables contain less calcium per serving than dairy products. The fiber in vegetables makes it harder for your body to extract and use the calcium in them — strange, but true.

Are soft drinks getting the best of you? Drinking carbonated soft drinks every day can zap the calcium out of your foods and supplements before it ever gets into your system. The phosphates in the soda bind with the calcium and magnesium, making them unusable. If you drink sodas regularly, increase your consumption of calcium. Doctors recommend menopausal women get 1,200 milligrams of calcium every day after age 50 (check with Table 4-1).

Many women find it easier to use calcium supplements than to get all the calcium they need from dairy products. With supplements, you know exactly how much calcium you're getting each day and most have the appropriate amounts of two other nutrients critical to bone building — vitamin D and magnesium. When choosing a supplement, avoid those made from oyster shell and dolomite. These supplements can be contaminated with toxic heavy metals. Calcium-carbonate antacids are one of the cheapest and easiest calcium supplements to find. As long as the calcium-carbonate antacid has no aluminum, it's safe to take every day. We personally prefer a calcium supplement that also contains vitamin D and magnesium, two other nutrients critical to healthy bone maintenance.

Women should get 400–600 milligrams of vitamin D and magnesium every day to maintain healthy bones. In other words, you should have about half as much vitamin D and magnesium every day as calcium. Magnesium prevents bone loss by playing an active role in bone growth. It also supports nerve cell communication (preventing wild mood swings), helps regulate blood pressure, and aids in muscle contraction. The last two functions help to prevent heart attacks. The heart is essentially one big muscle so magnesium helps keep the contractions regular. Also, magnesium seems to prevent spasms of the blood vessels, particularly in the arteries around the heart.

Calcium supplements with magnesium help prevent the constipation that some women experience when they take calcium supplements. Magnesium is a natural laxative and one of the main ingredients in milk of magnesia.

Vitamin K helps keep the body from cannibalizing bone for calcium by maintaining proper levels of calcium in the blood. Vitamin K also produces a protein used to build bone called *osteocalcin.* You can get vitamin K in green leafy vegetables like spinach and broccoli. You should get at least 100 micrograms of vitamin K a day. (Half a cup of broccoli has about 150 micrograms of vitamin K.)

Caffeine

Women who drink four or more cups of coffee a day increase their risk of fractures due to osteoporosis. Caffeine promotes bone loss by increasing the amount of calcium in your urine. Because coffee seems to have more caffeine than tea or colas, curbing your coffee habit is one of the best ways to reduce your caffeine intake in the quest for healthier bones. You can also switch to decaffeinated beverages.

Foods to watch

You know about the vast array of diets and dieting products available today to help you lose weight.

Be aware that high-protein foods and diets may not be good for your bones. Acids are sent into the bloodstream to help digest the protein, and your body hits the bone up for calcium to neutralize these acids. This leads to bone loss.

Women who eat a lot of red meat each week (5 servings or more) increase their risk of fractures by 20 percent. Vegetable proteins don't seem to cause the same responses as proteins from meats. So if you're going on a high protein diet, it's better to get your proteins from fish or vegetables.

Finding Out whether You Have Osteoporosis

Most women who have osteoporosis don't feel anything unusual — it's a silent disease. Unfortunately, most women find out they have low bone density only after they've had a fracture. Other women first notice it in the mirror — their posture seems poor, even when they stand up as straight as they can. Still other women have a chest x-ray for some unrelated reason and the doctor notices crushed vertebrae, indicating brittle bones.

One of the best ways to get a head's up on this disease is to have a bone-density screening, a painless, noninvasive test. You simply lie down on a padded table, (usually you don't even need to take your clothes off), and a machine passes over your body and records images. That's it!

To check out your bones, physicians concerned with prevention may recommend that you get a bone-density screening sometime before you're 40 and then routinely thereafter to measure bone mineral density (often abbreviated BMD) in two strategic locations — your spine and your hip.

Bone-density tests can help your doctor answer three important questions:

1. How much bone, if any, have you lost?
2. How quickly are you losing bone?
3. What's the best therapy to get your bones healthier and keep you from losing more bone?

The bone-density test produces a graphic image of your bone as well as statistics that compare your bones to healthy bones. You can find out how quickly you're losing bone by having these tests repeated every two or three years. The results of your bone-density test will guide your physician in choosing an appropriate therapy for bone loss, if one is needed.

Doing the DEXA

To measure bone density, most physicians use a test called a *dual energy x-ray absorptiometry,* or DEXA for short, which uses a fraction of the radiation a chest x-ray uses.

Preparing an image of your hip only takes a few minutes, and preparing an image of your spine only takes a few minutes more. The technician can see the results immediately, although you often receive your report a few days later. (They don't want the insurance company to think that the procedure isn't worth the money.)

The report shows colored images of your spine and hip reflecting different bone densities. The statistics that accompany the images compare your bone density to that of the average 35-year-old woman and to women your own age. (See the "Reading a DEXA report" sidebar nearby.)

When you begin losing bone (and everyone does), you need to figure out whether you're losing it slowly or quickly. Therefore, it's important to get a baseline test sometime between the ages of 35 and 40 and to continue to monitor your bone density throughout your life. Most doctors recommend that you check your bone density about every two years. You can compare the most current results to the previous results to determine the rate of loss (or gain).

Reading a DEXA report

The first thing you'll notice on the DEXA bone-density report is the colorful graphic image of your hip or spine. The technician generally tests both the spine and hip, and the reports for each are nearly identical; therefore, we walk through the spine report, and you can then apply this information to the hip report as well. The *lumbar vertebrae* (lower back) are analyzed for the spine test. The report you receive looks almost like an x-ray except it displays colors that correspond to different bone densities. Typically, a legend shows the color gradient going from low-density bone to high-density bone. This allows you to see exactly where the low-density areas are.

Statistics that compare your *bone mineral density* (BMD) measurements to those of 35-year-olds are displayed adjacent to the image. You may wonder why your measurements are compared to a 35-year-old woman's measurements. And who is this 35 year old that you're being compared to? Well, scientists have taken a large group of 35-year-old women, measured them and used the average bone densities as a standard of comparison. When they compare your bone density to this "standard," the difference is represented as a percentage. In other words, if your bones were half as dense as the average 35-year-old's, your statistics would read 50 percent; if your bones were the same, it would read 100 percent.

Suppose your comparison shows that your bones are within 85 percent of a 35-year-old. Is this terrible, or is it terrific? To determine if this percentage is statistically significant (something worth treating), the report includes a *T-score*.

For those of you who weaseled your way out of taking statistics, T-scores show how many standard deviations your score is from "normal." In this case, *normal* is the score of a healthy 35-year-old woman of your ethnic background. Negative T-scores aren't so good.

A T-score of –1, isn't too bad (unless you have already experienced unexplained fractures). Your doctor will probably diagnose you with *osteopenia*, which means you have low bone density (see Table 4-2 for the criteria used in diagnosing osteoporosis). If your T-score is –2.5 or lower, your doctor will probably diagnose you as having osteoporosis and recommend a course of treatment or some kind of dietary/fitness intervention.

If you're at high risk for osteoporosis due to genetics or life events, have your initial bone-density test during your early thirties, and have subsequent tests every two years after that.

Opting for another type of test

The DEXA bone-density measurement is probably the most commonly used procedure, but you or your doctor may opt for another procedure. Several devices work on the same principle as the DEXA bone scanner, including

- ✔ **Dual photon absorptiometry (DPA):** Introduced in the early 1980s, DPA was one of the first devices that could measure bone density in the spine and hip — the best bones to use as predictors of total body bone density. Earlier devices couldn't measure density in bone covered by heavy muscle, so they were restricted to testing the wrist and heel.

   This machine is a bit slower than today's DEXA — it takes about an hour to measure the hip and spine. Also, this machine isn't as precise as DEXA and can't measure small changes, so using it for comparisons is more difficult.

- ✔ **Quantitative computed tomography (QTC):** Also known as *CAT scans* or *CT scans,* QTCs can measure bone density anywhere in the body. The advantage of this procedure over the others is that it can accurately measure the center of each vertebra in the spine. DEXA measurement can only measure a certain type of vertebrae because other bones are in the way.

   CAT scans aren't typically used to measure a patient's bone density on a yearly basis because it exposes the patient to more radiation than the other techniques — and they're pretty expensive.

- ✔ **Ultrasound:** This test is sometimes used to measure bone density in the heel or kneecap. These machines are portable, so theoretically, more people can be screened using this quick, inexpensive bone-screening procedure. On the down side, this machine is limited to measuring bone density in *peripheral* sites — places other than the preferred spine and hip sites. If an ultrasound detects low bone density, you should have a follow-up DEXA test.

- ✔ **Urine tests:** As bone dissolves, some of the byproducts show up in urine. When performed every few months, urine tests can tell whether bone loss is increasing or decreasing.

   This test isn't an accurate diagnostic instrument for osteoporosis because you can have low bone density but be losing bone slowly. The test is generally used with patients on a treatment program for osteoporosis to monitor progress.

X-rays are *not* used to test for bone density because changes in the "whiteness" of the bone on the x-ray can't be detected until you've lost 30 percent of your normal bone mass. Clearly you want to take some action before you lose 30 percent of your bone mass.

Treating Osteoporosis

The first step in reducing bone loss is eliminating unhealthy habits (smoking and excessive alcohol use, for example) and picking up healthy habits (such as a healthful diet and an exercise program). Even the least invasive treatment programs, such as calcium supplements and increased exercise, can slow bone loss and improve bone density.

More aggressive treatment programs include atendronate sodium and/or hormone therapies. These programs can slow and even reverse bone loss. Many physicians recommend that women at high risk of osteoporosis begin hormone therapy during menopause. Estrogen levels need to be at least half of the level that they are at during a normal menstrual cycle to prevent bone loss. Some women who have lost a significant amount of bone may have testosterone added to their hormone regimen. Hormone therapy should be started early in menopause in addition to the other treatment programs.

Chapter 5

You Gotta Have Heart

*W*hen it comes to matters of the heart, men and women have their differences (but you already knew that, didn't you?). Many men have their first heart attack between the ages of 45 and 55, but women usually don't have heart trouble until after they reach menopause (at an average age of 51). And, if a woman has a heart attack during mid-life, she's more likely than a man to die from it. Why? One reason is that women have different symptoms than men. The crushing chest pains that warn men of heart attack aren't as common in women when they experience a heart attack. (The warning signs of heart attack for women are just a few of the many heart-healthy tips you can find in this chapter.)

In this chapter, we discuss heart attacks and many other types of cardiovascular disease. Your risk for cardiovascular disease increases after menopause because you lose the protective benefits of estrogen. (We don't discuss *congenital* heart problems in this chapter because these problems don't begin at menopause. They begin at birth.)

But you can keep your heart healthy even after menopause. And what would this chapter be if we just covered the bad news? We also discuss ways to keep your heart happy after the change — adopting a heart-healthy diet, getting a bit of exercise, and eliminating some bad habits.

Cardiovascular Disease and the Menopausal Woman

Estrogen, the female hormone produced in the ovaries, is good for your heart. *Estradiol,* the active form of estrogen, is the most beneficial form of estrogen, but (you guessed it) it's the type of estrogen that decreases as you become menopausal. (Chapter 2 is full of information about what your hormones do — check it out.)

Basically, estradiol is our secret weapon against all kinds of cardiovascular diseases. It's what every man wishes he had so that he could avoid the early onset of heart problems.

You may have heard that before age 80, women are about half as likely as men their age to have heart disease. This statement has led many people to perceive heart disease as largely a male problem. It isn't. Men do tend to develop heart problems about 10 years earlier than women, so on average, a woman has the heart of a man 10 years her junior. But just because men develop heart disease at an earlier age doesn't mean that heart disease isn't deadly for women. Just as many women as men die of heart disease each year.

Cardiovascular disease (disease of the heart and blood vessels) increases in women as estradiol levels decrease. After menopause, your risk of cardiovascular disease shoots way up. Between 45 and 65 years of age, men experience three times more heart attacks than women. But after age 65, watch out — women have more heart attacks than men.

We want to give you the total picture here, and unfortunately, that includes some info you may not want to hear. Of all the ways a menopausal woman can pass into the hereafter, cardiovascular disease is the most likely culprit. In fact, after menopause, you're ten times more likely to die from cardiovascular disease than from breast cancer.

For some reason, the word hasn't gotten out to women or their doctors. Heart disease kills more women each year than breast, ovarian, uterine, and cervical cancers combined. Also, diagnoses of heart disease and heart attacks are often delayed in women because the symptoms aren't recognized and taken seriously.

The term *cardiovascular disease* (CVD) encompasses conditions that affect your heart and blood vessels such as heart disease, heart attack, high blood pressure, coronary-artery disease, and stroke. All of these diseases restrict the flow of blood to the heart or brain.

Your Cardiovascular System

Understanding how your heart and blood vessels work reveals the role estrogen plays in your cardiovascular system. In its simplest form, your cardiovascular system consists of your blood vessels and that big pumping muscle you know as your heart (see Figure 5-1). Estrogen (in particular, the active form, estradiol) does a lot to keep your blood vessels and heart healthy and free from disease. The following list of ways estradiol protects you from getting an achy-breaky heart pulls together all the studies that have been done on estradiol and the cardiovascular system.

✔ It lowers your blood pressure by dilating blood vessels.

✔ It increases the good cholesterol and lowers the bad.

✔ It keeps platelets (part of your blood) from clotting too quickly.

✔ It acts like an antioxidant to keep fat deposits from forming on the walls of your arteries.

✔ It facilitates the release of a chemical that relaxes blood vessels, which helps reduce vessel spasms and increase blood flow.

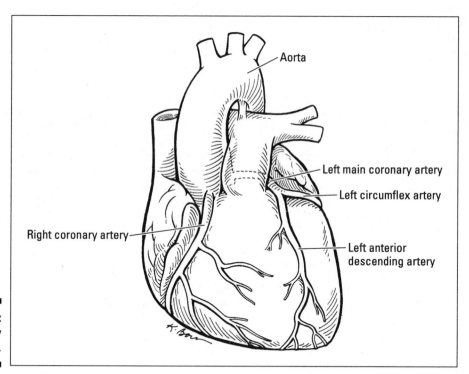

Figure 5-1:
The healthy heart.

Blood carries oxygen to the heart and picks up garbage on the way back. Fatty blood can wreak havoc on your cardiovascular system.

Looking at lipids or considering cholesterol

From the time you reach puberty to the time you start menopause, you probably have better cholesterol profiles than men of the same age. Women typically have higher levels of the good cholesterol (HDL) and lower levels of the bad cholesterol (LDL) than men during these years. But by the time you're menopausal, your LDL levels have risen and often exceed those of men your age.

Total cholesterol is not the total story for women. In men, higher levels of *total* cholesterol and heart disease go hand in hand. For women, the script is different. The *ratio* of LDL to HDL, as opposed to the sum of these two readings, is more important in predicting heart disease in women. The target ratio of LDL to HDL for women is 3.22 or less. The lower the ratio the better. But a woman's HDL level is even more important than her LDL-to-HDL ratio. HDL levels in healthy women are over 70 mg/dl. (That crazy looking unit of measure stands for *milligrams per deciliter,* but just remember it as the unit the medical folks tack onto cholesterol readings.)

The whole ball of wax that is cholesterol is broken down into various components:

- ✔ **Cholesterol:** At its basic level, *cholesterol* is fat — waxy, yellowish, oily fat. However, this fat (also known as a *lipid* in med speak) is critical to keeping your well-oiled body running. Your body uses cholesterol to build and repair cells and to produce hormones, such as estrogen and testosterone, vitamin D, bile (used to absorb fat), and myelin (coats the nerves). If your blood contains too much cholesterol, the cholesterol gets deposited with other crud on the inside of your blood vessels. Cholesterol travels through your bloodstream on the back of proteins, so the particles are named *lipoproteins* (get it? — lipid plus protein equals lipoprotein). Lipoproteins with more protein than fat are called high-density lipids (HDL), and those with more fat than protein are called low-density lipids (LDL).

- ✔ **High-density lipids (HDLs):** These lipids are called the "good" cholesterol because they help prevent the buildup of plaque. Because HDLs are mostly protein with just a little bit of fat, they can carry the extra bad cholesterol back to the liver so that the body can (literally) flush it away.

- ✔ **Low-density lipids (LDLs):** Also known as the "bad" cholesterol, LDLs are mostly fat and only a small amount of protein. At normal levels, they carry cholesterol from the liver to other parts of the body where it's needed for cell repair. When LDL cholesterol is too high, it adheres to the walls of the arteries and attracts other substances. The combined glob is called *plaque.*

- ✔ **Triglycerides:** In addition to the fat known as cholesterol, your blood contains this other type of fat in small quantities. Triglycerides have very little protein. They're almost pure fat, and the body uses them to store energy.

- ✔ **Total cholesterol:** This isn't literally another type of cholesterol. The term refers to a measure of the total amount of cholesterol in your blood.

To help separate the good cholesterol from the bad stuff in your mind, just remember **Lousy DeaL:** Low-density lipids (LDLs) are the "bad" cholesterol behind plaque formation.

You really don't need to eat *any* cholesterol after the age of one because your liver produces enough cholesterol on its own. Animal products such as meat, eggs, and dairy foods are especially high in cholesterol. Even though people don't need to eat these types of food to get enough cholesterol, most folks enjoy meat, cheese, birthday cake (which is full of butter and eggs), and other good stuff packed with cholesterol.

To find out the shape your blood is in, your doctor checks your cholesterol and triglyceride levels by taking a blood sample. The results, a *cholesterol profile* or *a lipoprotein analysis,* include your LDL, HDL, total cholesterol, and triglyceride levels. Using this information, your doctor can identify problems with your lipids and evaluate your risk of artherosclerosis.

The results from your cholesterol profile help you determine if your cholesterol and triglyceride levels are normal or off the charts. In Table 5-1, you can see what the National Institutes of Health have to say about healthy cholesterol and triglyceride levels. If your results are more like those in the third row of numbers, your doctor may want to talk to you about improving your diet or taking some medication.

Table 5-1	Cholesterol Ranges (mg/dl)		
Total Cholesterol	*HDL*	*LDL*	*Triglycerides*
Good < 200	> 60	< 130	< 150
Marginal 200–240	35–60	130–160	150–500
Bad > 240	< 35	> 160	> 500

Following the process and looking at the factors

We all know that you are what you eat, but diet isn't the only thing that controls your blood cholesterol. Exercise, insulin, obesity, and age also influence cholesterol levels.

Your genes probably have the biggest influence on your cholesterol profile. Marcia's mother, for example, nibbles on salads, avoids desserts, and rarely uses butter. Despite her low-fat eating habits, Mom's cholesterol profile is actually worse than Dad's profile — and he loves to eat cholesterol-intensive grilled cheese sandwiches and milk shakes with the grandchildren (when he's not snacking on a cream-of-something soup). It may not seem fair, but there you have it.

Regulating estrogen's role

Estradiol (the active type of estrogen) plays a major role in the way lipids are produced, managed, broken down, and eliminated from the body. Estradiol also seems to help dilate the blood vessels and keep them from having spasms. This may be part of the reason that women are prone to cardiovascular problems after menopause.

Natural estradiol is one thing, but hormone therapy is another when it comes to protecting your cardiovascular system. Take a look at Chapter 11 for more details on this subject, but here's the bottom line on hormones:

✓ **Combination hormone therapy:** Taking progesterone and estrogen increases a woman's HDL (good cholesterol) levels, but it also increases her LDL (bad cholesterol) levels and triglycerides.

✓ **Unopposed estrogen therapy:** Only women without a uterus should take estrogen alone. *Oral estrogen therapy* (without progesterone) increases HDL levels and decreases LDL levels. Unfortunately triglyceride levels tend to go up, which is not so good.

The *estradiol skin patch* when used without progesterone increases HDL and decreases LDL levels after about six months of use. More good news is that the patch also keeps triglycerides in check.

When it comes to blood cholesterol, unopposed estrogen therapy offers the best chance for improvement through hormone therapy. And the estradiol patches when used alone provide the most beneficial results to date. But only women who have had their uterus removed should take estrogen alone. Estrogen without progesterone raises the risk of endometrial cancer in women who have a uterus.

Connecting the dots between bad blood and cardiovascular disease

If your artery walls are injured (as a result of smoking, cocaine-usage, diabetes, or other factors), your body may react too aggressively in repairing the walls. White blood cells come to the rescue and bring cholesterol with them to patch over the damaged area. After a while, other stuff adheres to the spot and this patch becomes harder, like a callous. This harder stuff is called *plaque.* This is how bad habits or disease can lead to hardening of the arteries — what your doctor refers to as *atherosclerosis.*

Sometimes people have way too much LDL cholesterol and not enough HDL to carry it out of their bloodstream. When this happens, LDL cholesterol gets deposited on the artery walls and rots. (Antioxidants can prevent the rotting, which is one reason that nutritionists tell folks to get plenty of antioxidants if they want to be good to their hearts.) Other substances then collect with the rotting cholesterol to form plaque. This is how high cholesterol can lead to hardening of the arteries.

The latter process is a lot like the buildup that causes the drains in your kitchen sink to clog. Garbage goes down your sink every day, and every day, a little bit of gunk gets stuck on your pipes. Pretty soon the gunk buildup slows down the water as it moves through the pipes.

With time, calcium begins to form on the plaque, hardening the arteries. Now your arteries are narrowed and hardened, and blood has a hard time flowing to the heart. Just as the water backs up in your sink because of the clog, the blood backs up in your arteries when they become stopped up. Narrowing arteries can force your heart to pump harder to get the blood around your body. When your blood needs more pressure than normal, you have *hypertension* (high blood pressure).

Sometimes the plaque in your artery breaks off and gets lodged in a blood vessel, as shown in Figure 5-2. Imagine pouring clog-busting chemicals down your drain; except instead of dissolving the clog, the chemicals just loosen the gunk. Then the chunk o' gunk gets stuck in the curve of the pipe. When a piece of plaque gets stuck in a blood vessel, the area of heart muscle that gets fed by that vessel dies, and you have a heart attack.

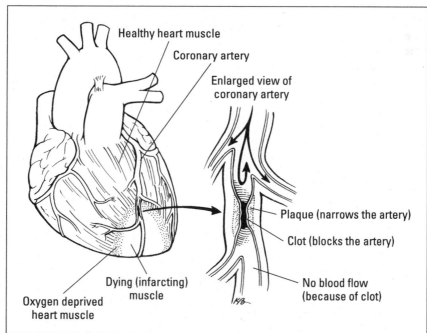

Figure 5-2: The thing to look at is the clog on the right. Your heart shouldn't look like this.

Understanding Cardiovascular Diseases

A whole family of diseases affects your cardiovascular system, and a lot of inbreeding goes on in this family. For example, high cholesterol can lead to hardening of the arteries. Hardening of the arteries can lead to heart attack or stroke as well as angina. Hypertension can lead to heart attack or stroke. It goes round and round and your risk of all of these conditions increases as your natural estrogen levels decline after menopause.

In this section, we introduce you to the members of the cardiovascular-disease family. Don't worry, we talk about preventing and treating unexpected visits from these conditions, too.

Containing coronary artery disease

Coronary artery disease (CAD) affects the blood vessels (the *coronary arteries*) that supply blood to your heart muscle. If these vessels are damaged, or if you have too much cholesterol in your blood, coronary arteries become narrowed or blocked by plaque as cholesterol and calcium buildup inside them. This process is called hardening of the arteries, or *atherosclerosis*. When the heart doesn't get enough oxygenated blood because of partially or totally blocked arteries, your heart muscle pays the price. The result is *coronary heart disease*. Coronary heart disease may cause angina (chest pain that we talk about in the "Avoiding angina" section later in this chapter) or a heart attack (check out the "Holding off heart attacks" section also found later in this chapter). Here's a depressing factoid: Nearly a million women in the United States develop coronary heart disease during the course of a year.

Women often underestimate the severity of their chest pains or don't realize that the chest pains are related to heart problems; therefore, they play down the symptoms to their physician. A couple of the reasons women give for not seeking help immediately are that they didn't want to inconvenience anyone and that they thought that heart disease was a guy thing.

Avoiding angina

To function properly, the heart muscle needs a constant supply of oxygen and nutrients delivered by the blood. If your veins or arteries become narrowed by fatty buildup in the artery walls (atherosclerosis), you may experience severe chest pain called *angina*. You feel pain because insufficient amounts of blood are getting through your veins into your heart muscle, and your heart is straining to pump enough blood to keep your body going strong.

Angina can also be caused by spasms in the blood vessels that block blood flow to the heart. Spasms can occur even if no blockages are present. Women are much more likely than men to suffer angina with no evidence of blockages.

Symptoms sometimes begin during physical activity or emotional stress. They typically last about ten minutes and go away after several minutes of rest. But many women experience chest pain while they're resting. This is typically triggered by spasms or an *arrhythmia* (irregular heartbeat).

Attention all women! Angina is a very common early warning sign of coronary artery disease (CAD). Because CAD is so lethal in women, heart specialists typically schedule further tests right away for women with severe chest pains. (For more on coronary artery disease, check out the "Containing coronary artery disease" section earlier in this chapter.)

Unfortunately, a survey studying how emergency-room doctors treated patients with severe chest pain showed that men received much more aggressive and quicker treatment than women. Also, men were twice as likely as women to be sent for *coronary arteriography* (a special test that looks at the coronary arteries) and bypass surgery after complaining of chest pain.

Holding off heart attacks

Menopausal and postmenopausal women are at an increased risk of heart attack (*myocardial infarction* in medicalese). Most women experience heart attacks after age 60, but heart disease may begin as early as the preteen years. Cholesterol accumulations have been found in girls as young as ten years old. These accumulations in young children, called *fatty streaks,* sometimes turn into more significant buildup later in life.

Blocked arteries often cause heart attacks. Either plaque breaks loose or a *blood clot* (a mass of solidified blood) blocks an artery cutting off blood supply to the heart. If the blockage remains in place for 5 to 10 minutes or more, the piece of the heart muscle fed by that artery begins to die.

Vessel spasms and arrhythmia are two additional causes of heart attacks, and evidence suggests that they're more common triggers of heart attack in women than in men. *Spasms* constrict your coronary arteries so blood can't get to the heart. Spasms can also cause plaque to break away from the vessel and get lodged in an artery, cutting off blood supply that way. *Arrhythmia,* or an irregular heartbeat, can mess up the pumping action of the heart and cut off blood supply as well.

Women often have different symptoms before a heart attack than men do. The symptoms are easy to overlook because they're often subtle and typical of many other, less serious problems. Often, women look back and say,

"Oh yeah, now that you mention it, I felt that way yesterday," after the heart attack has already occurred.

Pay attention to warning signs. As a woman, you may not feel the typical crushing, squeezing, heaviness, or burning chest pain that many men feel prior to a heart attack. Instead you may experience one or more of the following symptoms:

- ✔ Back pain
- ✔ Bloating
- ✔ Chest pain while resting
- ✔ Fatigue
- ✔ Heartburn or abdominal pain
- ✔ Jaw pain
- ✔ Joint pain
- ✔ Lightheadedness/fainting
- ✔ Shortness of breath
- ✔ Sweating

An unfortunate byproduct of a heart attack is a condition called ventricular fibrillation. *Ventricular fibrillation* refers to an irregular heartbeat that happens when the main pumping chambers of the heart, the *ventricles,* can't get coordinated; therefore, the blood can't get to the far reaches of the body.

Fending off hypertension

High blood pressure is another one of those health issues that's more likely to pop up as you get older. Until age 55, women usually have lower blood pressure than men. Between 55 and 65 years of age, women and men are about equal in the incidence of high blood pressure. After 65, more women than men have high blood pressure. So, just when you're dealing with all the symptoms connected with menopause, you may develop high blood pressure (your doctor may call it *hypertension*).

About half of all Caucasian women and three-quarters of African-American women over 50 have hypertension. For some reason, African-American women are more prone to hypertension than Caucasian women. Mexican-American women have about as high a chance of having hypertension as Caucasians, but Cuban-American and Puerto Rican women have lower incidence of hypertension.

No one knows why people develop high blood pressure. About 5 percent of the time, high blood pressure is caused by a condition such as diabetes or pregnancy, and it often can go away with treatment or resolution of the precipitating condition.

To visualize high blood pressure, think of blowing up a balloon. As you hold the balloon opening to your mouth and blow, the air in your mouth is under a great deal of pressure because you're trying to pass it through the small opening in the balloon. Now, think of your heart as your cheeks and your arteries as the balloon opening — the smaller the balloon opening, the more pressure in your cheeks as you try to blow. So, if your blood vessels get smaller due to cholesterol buildup, or whatever, your heart has to pump harder to pass the blood through these narrower openings. The result: Your blood pressure rises.

High blood pressure can lead to heart attack, kidney damage, bleeding in the retina behind your eyes, and stroke. For these reasons, having your blood pressure checked routinely after you reach 40 (or at any age) is critical.

Many women develop high blood pressure because of obesity. Fortunately, these women often can reduce their blood pressure dramatically by switching to a heart-healthy diet (see Chapter 18) and losing weight.

If you're not overweight, you may need to try some other types of intervention. Some women are able to regulate their blood pressure by reducing anxiety through meditation or other relaxation techniques. If these techniques don't work, medication may be the answer to getting your blood pressure under control. You may have to work with your doctor to find just the right type of drug and dosage. One drug may work for others but not for you. And, for some reason, drugs used to control blood pressure are more effective in men than women.

Staving off stroke

A stroke can occur for one of two reasons: either a blood clot blocks the flow of blood to your brain or a blood vessel in your brain ruptures. In either case, oxygen-rich blood can't get to the brain to nourish it. The problems a stroke cause depend upon the location and severity of the stroke, but speech problems, physical weakness, paralysis, and permanent brain damage are all possible stroke complications. Many stroke victims go through rehabilitation programs that restore full or partial function to the affected areas of the body.

Here are the symptoms associated with strokes:

- Difficulty talking or understanding speech
- Dizziness
- Loss of vision, particularly in just one eye
- Unexplained numbness or weakness in the face, an arm, a leg, or one side of your body

A *transient ischemic attack* (TIA) is like a mini-stroke. During a TIA, blood flow to the brain is interrupted (usually by a blood clot). The symptoms of a TIA usually last only 10 to 20 minutes and end when blood flow returns to normal. At worst, the symptoms of a TIA last 24 hours; symptoms of a stroke can last a lifetime. If you have any of the symptoms listed in conjunction with the stroke discussion, see a doctor.

Pay attention to TIAs because they can be early warning signs of an impending stroke. Half of the people who have a TIA suffer a stroke within a year.

Cardiovascular Disease Risk Factors for Women

Many of the risk factors for cardiovascular-disease-related complications are more risky for women (particularly menopausal women) than men, but many are risk factors for both men and women — even men and women who seem to be in good health.

- **Alcohol:** Women don't produce as much of a specific enzyme used to break down alcohol (*alcohol dehydrogenase*) as men do. So women tend to feel the buzz from alcohol earlier than men, and alcohol stays in their systems longer. Three or four drinks a day will cause a noticeable rise in blood pressure. (We outline the dangers of high blood pressure in the nearby "Fending off hypertension" section.) In large doses, alcohol acts like a poison and kills heart tissue.

- **Cholesterol:** Low HDL levels and a high LDL-to-HDL ratio increase a woman's risk for cardiovascular disease. After menopause, most women's HDL levels drop a little bit. A bigger change takes place in your LDL level. As women age, LDL levels keep rising — especially between the ages of 40 and 60. So your HDL and LDL levels and your LDL-to-HDL ratio are usually worse as you age.

- **Cocaine use:** Cocaine and its relative — crack — are seriously dangerous drugs. Cocaine, whether snorted, smoked, or injected, can cause serious damage to women's arteries and heart. Here are a few conditions cocaine and crack use can cause: spasms in the coronary arteries, restricted oxygen flow to the heart, and arrhythmia. If a woman has a previous coronary-related condition such as a *mitral valve prolapse* (heart murmur), cocaine can cause sudden death.

- **Diabetes:** High blood pressure, excessive weight, and inactivity can lead to adult-onset diabetes in women. Although adult-onset diabetes isn't real common, it's very serious for menopausal women. Diabetes can cause a host of other problems, one of which is an increased risk of heart disease. Here's the scoop on women, diabetes, and cardiovascular disease:

- Women over 45 (menopausal women) are twice as likely as men their age to develop diabetes.

- Women with diabetes are more than five times more likely to have some type of coronary "event" (we're not talking about a gala here; we're talking about a heart attack, angina, and so on) than women without diabetes.

- Women with diabetes are four times more likely to die of a heart attack. In fact, 80 percent of all people who suffer from diabetes die of heart attacks.

Fortunately, adult onset diabetes can often be prevented or controlled through weight loss, exercise, and a healthy diet.

✔ **Excessive weight:** If you weigh 20 percent or more than your target weight, you're overweight. (Chapter 18 has a chart you can use to determine where you are in relations to your target weight.) For example, if your *target weight* (how much people your height and build should weigh) is 125, you're overweight if you weigh 150 pounds or more. Excessive weight increases your risk of high blood pressure, heart disease, stroke, and even diabetes. Because excessive weight leads to many diseases and complications, it only makes sense that losing the excessive weight can lower your risk for many diseases and complications. Excessive weight is a huge and growing problem (no pun intended) — more than one-third of all White women and half of all Black women in the United States are overweight.

✔ **High blood pressure:** High blood pressure can lead to heart attacks and stroke because it stresses out the blood vessels. Stress on your blood vessels can constrict the arteries and cause plaque to separate from the vessel wall and clog your arteries.

✔ **Inactivity:** For women, inactivity is the most common risk factor for cardiovascular disease. Most women never had the time or chance to incorporate a "workout" into their busy schedules. Chauffeuring children and performing household chores, intermingled with a 40 to 50 hour workweek, often leaves women with no time or desire to take a walk or regularly attend an exercise class. Husbands and children (aren't they precious?) may question how you can waste an hour on an activity that doesn't directly benefit them or the household. Well, the fact is that you must make the time (just like your husband or kids do) for physical activity. Physical activity is not a waste of time — it lowers a woman's risk of heart problems by a whopping 50 percent. And keep in mind that half of all women die of cardiovascular disease. Take a look at Chapter 19 for some ideas on increasing your activity level.

✔ **Personality:** Many people believe that too much stress results in high blood pressure and heart attacks. Whether you're talking monkeys or people, the research indicates that it's a control thing, not a just a stress thing. Women (and monkeys) who feel in control of their lives are much less likely to have heart disease. Cholesterol profiles are also much better for women who feel in control of their jobs, lives, or homes. When you feel out of control, you're more likely to feel cynical or hostile, or you may feel sorry for yourself. Researchers have also linked these personality traits to a higher incidence of heart disease.

✔ **Smoking:** Cigarette smoking triples your risk of heart attack and angina. Even women who smoke less than five cigarettes a day double their risk of heart disease. When you inhale smoke, your heart beats faster, your blood vessels constrict, and your circulation slows down. The nicotine in cigarettes promotes blood clots (which can lodge in your arteries to cause heart attacks or stroke). Smokers also have a greater risk of high blood pressure and emphysema.

Being Smart about Your Heart

Eating a healthy diet, watching your weight, exercising routinely, avoiding unhealthy habits, and getting annual medical examinations are the best ways to prevent cardiovascular problems.

Weighing an ounce of prevention

Keeping your blood clean and lean really helps prevent hardening of the arteries, which is the source of many serious problems. Controlling your cholesterol boils down to eliminating unhealthy habits (smoking, drinking too much alcohol, using recreational drugs, and so on), sticking to a healthy diet (check out Chapter 18), and exercising five days a week for a half-hour (turn to Chapter 19).

If you're not able to control your cholesterol through lifestyle changes, you and your doctor can consider alternatives. A variety of medications are available today that can lower your cholesterol.

But many people develop hypertension even though their cholesterol levels are terrific. Doctors always seem to check your blood pressure as soon as you step in the door. So keep those doctor appointments and, if your blood pressure is high, seek help. Your doctor will work with you to find the right medication for you, but you're the one who has to take it every day if it's going to work.

Routine checkups (that means at least once a year) with your internist and gynecologist should prevent cardiovascular problems from sneaking up on you.

Treating what ails you

If you maintain regular appointments and seek help when you feel any weird happenings in your heart (like palpitations or pain), you should be pretty safe. Of course, you have to follow the advice given to you by professionals when problems are detected. If you have high blood pressure, you need to take your medication. Even though you usually have no symptoms with hypertension, not taking your medication can cause trouble — same goes for cholesterol. Many people have no symptoms when their cholesterol is high, but if they go untreated, faulty cholesterol levels can cause a world of problems.

Today, a variety of medications are available to treat these conditions. Sometimes you and your doctor will have to experiment a bit to find out which medicines work for you, but the effort is worth it because the reward is a prolonged life.

Chapter 6

Vaginal and Urinary Changes

*I*f you think it's difficult talking to your mom about menopause, envision talking to her about the vaginal and urinary problems associated with the change. Probably not going to happen? You're not alone. Many women live with pain and discomfort because they're too embarrassed to discuss these problems with anyone — not even their family members, friends, or doctors.

Someday, you may notice that your vagina doesn't seem to be performing its lubricating duties like it used to when you're about to engage in sex. Or maybe sex is becoming a bit uncomfortable. Your private parts may be dry, and you may experience itching around your vulva or in your vagina, a watery vaginal discharge, or a burning sensation when you tinkle. The medical term for this is *atrophic vaginitis,* or *vaginal atrophy* in more common terms.

Vaginal and urinary issues are not unique to menopausal women — some women experience vaginal dryness during sex long before they're menopausal, and other women who have been menopausal for several years have no problems with vaginal dryness. Some women experience vaginal irritation only temporarily; others find it gets worse with age. It's a very individual thing.

If you live long enough, without hormone therapy or some type of treatment, your vaginal lining is going to thin and become drier, but you may never experience any of the symptoms, pain, or discomfort. You may never even know that it's happening. Some women notice dryness during sex or itching that lasts a few months while their bodies adjust to the lower estrogen levels. Other women may experience discomfort during sex at first and then more intense symptoms as time goes on. If you do experience discomfort, you don't have to simply put up with it — many treatments are available.

Your urinary tract and your female organs are located next to each other, and both systems rely on estrogen to function properly. These two facts explain why problems can arise in both systems during the change and why changes in your vagina may affect your urinary tract.

Doc, Can We Talk?

Before you can do anything about urinary-tract or vaginal problems, you have to have a doctor diagnose your condition. Many problems exhibit symptoms that have nothing to do with menopause, so seeing a medical expert is a good idea.

You may think that talking to your doctor about painful sex or problems with your plumbing is embarrassing, but get over it. Your doctor has heard it all before. In fact, medical books tell doctors that patients underreport these problems because they're too embarrassed to talk about urinary and vaginal matters. Doctors are supposed to ask you about them, but they may not, so you need to bring up the subject.

Here are some tips for talking to your doctor about your symptoms:

✔ **Keep a diary:** You need to plan ahead for your visit to the doctor. If you experience vaginal or urinary-tract pain, keep track of when it hurts, where it hurts, the presence or absence of discharge, the color of the discharge, and any other details. If you experience urine leakage, write down what time you tinkled, how much urine was involved (use any measure you're comfortable with — cups, ounces, teaspoons, whatever — and let the doctor do the conversion), and what triggered the accident. (Did you lose it when you were laughing, exercising, sneezing, or watching TV?) Also note any type of discomfort and the level of pain.

✔ **Be specific:** When you discuss matters with your doctor, don't just say that you're uncomfortable "down there" and then lift your eyebrows to make your point. Tell the doc what symptoms you're experiencing.

✔ **Be persistent:** If the doctor's response isn't helpful — "That's normal for women your age" — press him on the issue to get the advice and help you need to deal with the problem. Just because "it's normal" doesn't mean that it can't be helped.

Vaginal Atrophy and Other Issues

Many women fear that the natural result of menopause is that their vagina dries out, shrivels up, and becomes a sexual wasteland. Well, that doesn't have to happen. In fact, *less than half* of all postmenopausal women complain of vaginal dryness or other symptoms of vaginal atrophy.

Who came up with the term *vaginal atrophy?* The term *atrophy* makes you think of stagnant, dead things, doesn't it? When we hear *atrophy,* we think of those plump little worms that get stranded on a sidewalk after a rainstorm and end up dried out and dead. Look up the word *atrophy* in the dictionary — it means "wasting away" and "failure to grow because of lack of nutrition." But vaginal dryness isn't an insurmountable problem at all, and we're here to tell you how to deal with it. Don't worry — your fate isn't linked to the fate of that poor little worm on the sidewalk.

Vaginal changes that accompany menopause don't have to make you uncomfortable or make sex unappealing. You have many ways at your disposal to keep your little flower pliable and moist so that sex can continue to be enjoyable. All menopausal women experience vaginal changes, but you can reduce the unwanted side effects.

What it is and what it isn't

We're going to start by describing what vaginal atrophy is not. It's not a condition that occurs only in women after menopause, and it doesn't mean your vagina is going to shrivel up and blow away.

So what is *vaginal atrophy?* Glad you asked. Because estrogen keeps your vagina moist and elastic, loss of estrogen can cause it to become drier, thinner, and less elastic. The downturn in estrogen production can also cause your vagina to shrink slightly in terms of width and length.

An atrophic vagina has lost some of its plumpness and firmness because the lining has thinned, and it doesn't have the furrows and folds typical of a fertile vagina. (Yes, this is one case in which wrinkles are a sign of youth.) The vagina appears red instead of pink. Also, with less mucous, the vagina becomes less acidic, so it's easier for bacteria to grow, which causes the watery discharge some women experience.

Talk to your doctor about vaginal changes if you experience discomfort. Dryness and other vaginal-atrophy-related symptoms may prompt you to avoid sex just when you have more time for it. Don't be embarrassed to bring it up — your doctor knows of plenty of ways to fix this one.

What lower estrogen means for your vagina

Estrogen bathes the vagina (and your urinary tract), keeping the tissue lubricated and flexible. Estrogen is the secret behind keeping the female organs working like a well-oiled machine.

Here's what the relative lack of estrogen that menopause brings about can mean to you:

✔ Your vagina becomes more susceptible to tears or damage from friction.

Sexually transmitted diseases have an easier time invading your body through tears than through an intact lining. So, step up your protection after menopause. Also, because tearing your vagina is easier after menopause, watch the rough stuff.

✔ As vaginal tissues lose their elasticity, your vagina may become less pliant and sometimes smaller. Sex may be less enjoyable if you don't intervene with some type of therapy.

✔ Your vagina may not get as lubricated during sexual arousal as it did before menopause, so intercourse may be painful if you don't use a lubricant.

✔ Vaginal mucous keeps your vagina an acidic kind of place. This acidic environment destroys much of the bacteria introduced into the area (through sex or wiping after you go to the bathroom). When your production of vaginal mucous tails off, infections find it easier to grow in your vagina. After menopause, you become more susceptible to vaginal bacteria, so you can develop *bacterial vaginosis* (inflammation of the vagina caused by bacterial infection).

What to do about it

For some women, the easiest way to prevent or slow down the progress of vaginal atrophy (and probably the most enjoyable one) is to practice regular sexual activity. Sexual activity increases blood circulation and lubrication and promotes vaginal elasticity. If you don't have a sexual partner, masturbation provides the same benefits.

If dryness inhibits your sexual desire, try one of the many lubricants available over the counter. Some of the lubricants are for use during sexual activity; others act like a moisturizer and cause your vagina to absorb water. Some women also find that vitamin E relieves dryness. Break open a capsule and apply the oil directly to your vagina.

Applying estrogen cream to the vagina also provides relief from the pain and itching associated with vaginal dryness. Your best bet is to use these medications as prescribed by your physician.

Vaginal estrogen creams seem more effective for relieving discomfort due to dryness than oral hormone treatments. Although most of the estrogen stays in your vagina, some is absorbed into your bloodstream. However, doctors usually prescribe such a low dosage for this problem that using a vaginal estrogen cream shouldn't substantially increase your risk of endometrial cancer or breast cancer like oral estrogen does. In fact, vaginal creams are often prescribed for women who don't want to take hormones orally because they're at higher risk of endometrial or breast cancer.

As with hormone therapy (HT) and estrogen pills, you need a prescription from your doctor for these creams.

By the way, you can use a lubricant during sex in addition to the estrogen cream to keep things slippery.

Before we change subjects, here's one last tip: Drinking plenty of water keeps your entire body hydrated, including your vagina. Think of yourself as an athlete in training and follow an athlete's regimen: Drink more water. Drink less alcohol and coffee.

Hold It! We Need to Talk about Urinary Problems

A healthy urinary tract depends on healthy tissue and toned muscle around the plumbing. About 40 percent of women between the ages of 45 and 64 have urinary-tract problems, which mainly take the form of *incontinence* (inability to hold back urine). You may never have a urinary-tract problem, but if you do, you'll know the basics. In this chapter, we arm you with the information you need to know.

Urinary-tract problems are no longer kept in the closet as they once were. Everyday, it seems a new actor appears on a TV commercial confessing his or her problem. Many products are available to help control or eliminate urinary disorders so that you can enjoy all the activities you've always participated in. Ask you doctor about appropriate courses of treatment.

Your *urinary tract* moves liquid waste from your kidneys, through your bladder, and out to the toilet. For the most part, it consists of your kidneys, bladder, *ureter* (the duct that carries urine from the kidney to the bladder), and urethra. But never mind the technicalities, the relevant fact is that urinary-tract conditions are more common in women after menopause.

Bet you didn't know this: The end of the *urethra* (the little tube that your tinkle flows from) is more dependent on estrogen than any other part of your urinary tract. After menopause, when estrogen has been low for a period of time, that tube can become inflexible. Simultaneously, the collagen and connective tissue (the fleshy stuff) around your urethra that supports your plumbing gets thinner. So two problems can occur:

✔ With less flexibility and thinner tissue in and around your urethra, you're more likely to get some microscopic tearing that makes it easier for bacteria to enter the urethra. Therefore, urinary-tract infections (UTIs) can get started more easily.

> ✔ The urethra has a harder time sealing itself using pressure, so you may leak or dribble urine when you least expect it and have instances of incontinence.

Nearly one of every six women over 45 develops one of these urinary-tract problems. So don't feel embarrassed when you talk to your doctor. These problems are quite common and very treatable. But infections only become worse with time, so go to the doctor right away if you think you've got problems with your plumbing.

Take a look at the "Doc, Can We Talk?" section earlier in this chapter for recommendations on recording your symptoms in preparation for your visit to the doctor. For urinary-tract problems, you can talk to either your gynecologist or primary-care physician. Your doctor will refer you to a specialist if needed, but most of the time, a gynecologist or primary-care physician can handle these issues. We're not here to diagnose your problems, but in the following sections, we tell you a bit about each of these conditions and what your doctor might do about them.

Tracking urinary-tract infections

A whole slew of urinary-tract infections (UTIs) are out there, and they can affect areas of your bladder, kidneys, and so on. One thing all UTIs have in common is that they're mainly caused by bacteria entering your plumbing from your urethra.

The most common UTI, *cystitis,* affects your bladder. Women are more prone to bladder infections than men because we wipe after we use the toilet. That's right — just tidying up leads to problems. Wiping can sweep germs from your feces (bowel movements) into your urethra. These bacteria (especially E. coli) can travel all the way to your bladder (or further into your kidneys) and create an infection. (That's why you should follow your mother's advice — wipe from front to back).

Frequent or vigorous sex can harm the delicate tissue of the vulva and outer urethra, which in turn allows bacteria into the body causing urinary-tract infections. Peeing immediately after sex helps you avoid UTIs.

Getting to a diagnosis

If you have a urinary-tract infection, it usually starts with a burning sensation or pain when urinating accompanied by urgency, frequency, or both. (*Urgency* refers to feeling like your bladder is so full its about to burst and you can't make it to the bathroom. *Frequency* is that feeling that you have to go to the bathroom constantly.)

If you have a UTI, you may find yourself rushing to the bathroom, releasing just a trickle of urine, and then a short time later, feeling as if you have to go again. This pattern is especially irritating at night. Repeatedly waking up to shuffle off to the bathroom can leave you exhausted.

You may also notice that your urine is cloudy, has blood in it, or smells worse than usual. If the infection is in your kidneys, you may have a fever, chills, back pain, nausea, or vomiting.

Urgency, frequency, and pain related to peeing are also symptoms of other conditions. If you experience any or all of these symptoms, make an appointment with your medical advisor. You'll have to do the tinkle-in-a-cup routine so that the professionals can examine your urine to determine whether you have a UTI or some other condition. The tests your doctor may run include

- ✔ **Urinalysis:** The doc examines the urine under a microscope for white blood cells (which indicate an infection), bacteria, and so on.
- ✔ **Urine culture:** Your doctor sends your urine sample to a laboratory to find out exactly what type of bacteria is present.

Trying some treatments

Treatment usually includes a short course of antibiotics and directions to drink plenty of fluids.

Drinking several glasses of unsweetened cranberry juice every day also helps your recovery from a bladder infection. Cranberry juice makes urine more acidic, and thereby making it more difficult for bacteria to grow.

Don't use cranberry juice as an alternative to visiting your doctor if you think you may have a urinary-tract infection. Some dangerous conditions can develop if a urinary tract is left untreated.

Covering interstitial cystitis

Interstitial cystitis (IC) is often overlooked or misdiagnosed as a urinary-tract infection because the symptoms are so similar.

IC is rare, yet nearly a million women suffer from it each year in the United States. It can occur in women who have reached menopause, but some women also develop IC in their twenties or thirties.

No one knows what causes IC, but some have theorized that frequent bladder infections that cause the bladder to attack itself may cause the condition. Or perhaps an unrecognized bacterium attacks the bladder lining. Some medical professionals wonder aloud whether there's a link between hormones and IC.

We've mentioned that tissues in the bladder and throughout the urinary tract rely on estrogen. Well, the nerve-endings do too. When estrogen bathes these nerve endings during your reproductive years, you don't notice any sensation in your bladder until it's quite full because estrogen keeps your sensory threshold high. But, when your estrogen levels are reduced during perimenopause and menopause, your pain threshold is lowered and you become more sensitive in your bladder area. Here are more clues that suggest a possible role for hormones in connection with IC:

✔ The average age of an IC sufferer is 42.

✔ Premenopausal women who have IC seem to have recurrences during the part of the menstrual cycle when estrogen levels are falling.

Getting to a diagnosis

Interstitial cystitis is a specific type of bladder infection. Bacteria cause most bladder infections (bladder infections are known generically as *cystitis*), but if you have IC, your doctor won't find any bacteria when he analyzes your urine sample. It's not surprising then that antibiotics don't help. A lot of the symptoms of IC are similar to those of a bacterial bladder infection; these symptoms include frequent urination (especially at night), sudden urge to urinate, and pain that becomes worse as the bladder fills up. Sometimes the pain, which can get very intense during urination, subsides after urination. The symptoms may go away from time to time. It's all quite mysterious.

Sometimes the pain is pretty generalized and occupies your entire pelvic area. You may feel pressure, tenderness, or pain in your bladder and the area around your bladder. If you're still menstruating, the pain may get worse just before your periods. You may also have pain during intercourse.

Diagnosing IC isn't easy. In their search for a cause of your symptoms, doctors initially go through a process of elimination, testing for UTIs and other conditions. After they eliminate these other possible causes, docs may take a peak at your bladder by inserting a scope up through your urethra into your bladder (this is called a *cystoscopy*) to look for scarring or microscopic tears on the walls inside your bladder.

Trying some treatments

The treatment options range from the least invasive — modifying your diet — to the most invasive — bladder surgery to repair the walls or remove the entire bladder.

Some women find that eliminating certain foods from their diet helps relieve bladder irritation. These foods include alcohol, coffee, tobacco, sharp cheeses, artificial sweeteners, preservatives, and acidic foods. Dyes used in food and medicines have also been found to irritate the bladder or cause bladder spasms.

Between modifying your diet and having surgery, you may find success with some medications: A drug called Elmiron repairs some of the damage on the walls of the bladder, and mild analgesic narcotics can manage the pain.

Antibiotics are ineffective in treating an IC. Women misdiagnosed with a urinary-tract infection find that the antibiotics prescribed for that condition do little to help relieve the symptoms of IC.

Encountering incontinence

Three-year-olds have a hard time "holding it" when they don't recognize the signal telling them that they have to tinkle until it's too late. Later in life (after babies, surgery, and menopause) some women again have trouble "holding it," but for different reasons. Sometimes, your body doesn't follow the orders your brain calls out.

When you can't hold back urine, or urine leaks out when you don't want it to, you may be *incontinent*. Lower levels of estrogen contribute to reduced muscle tone in the urethra, so you can lose bladder control. Wear and tear on muscles from bearing children or surgery can make the problem even worse.

The urethra (the tube through which urine flows from the bladder out of your body) is controlled by having more pressure around the urethral tube than in the bladder, keeping it closed. Estrogen helps increase muscle tone that leads to increased pressure, which prevents leakage. With lower estrogen levels, the muscle fibers lose their flexibility. The urethra has a hard time making a nice tight seal where it connects to the bladder.

Getting to a diagnosis

Incontinence comes in a couple of varieties:

- ✔ **Stress incontinence:** Urine leaks when you laugh or sneeze or cough. Many women whose pelvic muscle tone is shot because of bearing children or having surgery suffer stress incontinence.

  The *stress* in *stress incontinence* has nothing to do with psychological pain you may or may not be feeling; it refers to the stress in your abdomen. When you cough or laugh, you create pressure in your abdomen, which puts pressure on the bladder, causing the bladder pressure to become greater than urethral pressure. So laughing and coughing set off a chain reaction that ends in leakage.

  About a third of the women who suffer from stress incontinence are premenopausal. After menopause, it can get worse.

- ✔ **Urge incontinence:** A less common type of incontinence. With urge incontinence, you feel a tremendous urge to urinate, but before you can get to the bathroom, you begin leaking. You get "caught short" because you just can't make it to the bathroom fast enough.

Spasms in your bladder cause this type of incontinence. Urge incontinence is usually caused by a more serious medical problem like a herniated disk in your back, *fibroids* (little, noncancerous wads of tissue), nerve damage, or even bladder cancer. Contact your doctor right away so he or she can check out this condition.

Trying some treatments

See your doctor if you experience any type of incontinence. Incontinence may be a symptom of another medical condition, and treating the symptom may not be the best way to treat the whole disease.

Incontinence due to weakened muscles in the pelvic floor can be treated with *Kegel exercises,* which strengthen the muscles around your urethra. If you went to childbirth classes, you may have heard of these exercises. Well, Kegels are as useful in menopause as they were after childbirth.

Strengthening the muscles supporting the urethra keeps you from leaking urine when you laugh, cough, or exercise. Kegel exercises also can help you improve the muscle tone in your *pubococcygeous* (PC) muscle — the muscle you use to stop urine from flowing.

The biggest problem with Kegels is that most women aren't taught the right way to do them, so they don't get the full benefit. The nearby "Kegel in three easy steps" sidebar starts your Kegel program off on the right foot.

Kegels can improve muscle tone, but they don't strengthen thinned tissue. If thinning tissue is the cause of incontinence, surgery may be the appropriate treatment.

Some other methods you can use to handle incontinence caused by weakened muscles include

- **Pads:** These pads are similar to the pads you wear during your menstrual period, and they function the same way — the pad absorbs leaked urine, and you change a used pad when you go to the bathroom.

  Gel-affixed, foam pads are also available. These little devices are either inserted like a tampon or worn over the opening of the urethra. You have to change them after urinating. This type of pad is most useful for women whose incontinence problem is primarily limited to certain activities such as exercise.

- **Silicone caps:** Silicone-rubber caps inserted into the urethra are now available and seem to reduce leakage by about 50 percent.

- **Teflon or collagen injections:** Some doctors are currently performing these procedures. The injected Teflon or collagen strengthens the tissues

Kegel in three easy steps

Every time you go to the bathroom, end the outing with a series of Kegel exercises. Although medical professionals usually say you only need do these exercises three times each day, you won't have to tax your memory if you just do them every time you urinate. If you follow this advice, you'll ensure that you're exercising routinely and frequently — two requirements for successfully strengthening the pubococcygeous (PC) muscle, which helps you stop urine from flowing. Here are the three steps to a stronger PC:

1. While you're urinating, squeeze the muscle you use to stop the flow of urine. Now that you've found your PC muscle, you're ready for the workout.

2. Squeeze the PC muscle for 3 seconds (one one-thousand, two one-thousand, three one-thousand) and then relax for 5 seconds. Try to squeeze only your PC muscle, keeping your thigh, abdomen, and buttocks muscles relaxed. Squeezing the other muscles actually works against the exercise because it creates pressure above the urethra, which makes it difficult to squeeze the PC muscle. Do this exercise five times every time you go to the bathroom.

3. Work up to holding each squeeze for 10 seconds and relaxing for 5 seconds in between squeezes. Continue doing five of these each time you go to the bathroom.

After 6 to 8 weeks, you should notice an improvement in your ability to control the flow of your urine. Practice while you're actually urinating to see if you can completely stop the flow.

around the urethra or bladder neck by making them thicker. You normally need multiple injections.

✔ **Vaginal cones:** This approach uses little weights (vaginal cones) to strengthen muscles related to controlling urine flow. You insert a tampon-like cone into your vagina and hold it there. The goal is to gradually increase the weight and the amount of time you hold the cone in place.

Talk to your doctor about these solutions and others (like electrical stimulation and vaginal urethral rings). Medications are available that inhibit bladder contractions, increase the fortitude of the bladder lining, or relax smooth muscle in both the urethra and bladder — all of which can help curb symptoms of incontinence. These medications include probanthine, flavoxate, oxybutynin, and imipramine — all of which control bladder spasms. As always, medications have side effects.

If your sleep is interrupted by incontinence, you restrict the amount of fluids you drink after dinner. Be sure to drink enough fluid during the day to make up for the curfew.

Chapter 7

Surfaces and Sinuses: Your Skin, Hair, and Nasal Cavities

- -

In This Chapter

▶ Ironing out the hormone-induced wrinkles and other skin changes

▶ Blowing the whistle on sinus problems

▶ Putting a cap on thinning hair

- -

No, you're not going crazy or losing your mind if you think that your skin has gotten drier over the years. Face it — dry skin happens. And it may be related to menopause. Depending on which scientists you believe, the sags and wrinkles in your face may or may not be due to lower levels of estrogen. Don't worry — we give you both sides of the story in this chapter.

How are your sinuses doing? Do you seem to have a runny nose more often since you turned 40? Guess what? This annoyance is tied to menopause as well. And, if you're like us, as a child, you watched an aunt or grandma in total amazement, wondering how that one hair on her chin got so long. Does grandma have to shave? Read on to find out why the hair on your head seems to migrate to your chin after the change.

We'll be the first ones to admit that no one is going to win a Nobel prize for discovering a pill to relieve the conditions described in this chapter. In the grand scheme of things, these conditions may be mosquito bites in relation to the other issues that women face during and after menopause. But they're really annoying, and they vex our vanity! So it's nice to know why they happen and what you can do about them. That's what this chapter is for.

Getting the Skinny on Skin

Marcia has been working out for years. Her motivation has always been the vivid memory of her fifth-grade teacher's flabby upper arm swinging back and forth as she wrote the assignments on the blackboard. Thirty children snickered as the wobble of loose flesh seemed to move to a rhythm all its own.

The fear of children snickering at her arms has kept Marcia jogging and lifting weights on a daily basis. But she'll never forget the time she looked down as she was running to see the top of her *forearm* jiggling. Oh the horror — how could that be? There's no fat there! As Marcia looked at her arm more closely, she realized that it wasn't fat that was jiggling; it was her *skin!* Her skin is no longer tight on her arms; it has loosened to the point that it wobbles as she runs. Fortunately, Marcia's vision is so bad now that, if she doesn't wear her glasses when she runs, she doesn't see the sagging skin jiggle.

Usually, during perimenopause (the years leading up to menopause) and menopause, you're on a heightened state of alert, looking for the changes you know are happening. Some of the changes include extra laugh lines or crow's feet around your eyes. You may also notice dry skin or dry scalp that you never had before.

Making the skin and hormone connection

Menopause (more specifically the associated decline of estrogen levels) probably accelerates many of the little annoying changes that accompany aging. But separating the skin changes due to low estrogen from those that come as a result of being on this planet for a long time can be difficult. Think about it. Forty plus years of gravity is going to contribute to sagginess. No matter whether you're a woman or a man, your skin has been fighting gravity's weight ever since you could sit upright. By the time you approach your seventies, you're left with jowls instead of cheeks and a "gobbler" instead of a nice, tight neck.

Placing blame for skin woes

Estrogen plays a role in the great skin caper. The collagen and elastin fibers that keep your skin supple, pliant, and nicely molded to your frame slowly deteriorate as the active form of estrogen declines. The deterioration of collagen and elastin fibers leaves room for the wrinkles. Wrinkles (creases in your skin) show up where muscles contract. For example, when you smile, several facial muscles pull tight, forming one or more lines in the skin adjacent to your mouth. With age, these lines stay behind even when you're not smiling.

Other wrinkles resemble straight or branched lines finely etched all over the weakened skin. These wrinkles are also the result of the double dip of low estrogen levels and aging.

The fatty layer under your skin disappears over time as well, and your skin loses its flexibility — which leads to the saggy skin Marcia watches flapping on her arms as she runs. If your skin were clothes, you'd probably go to the tailor to have it taken in. (In fact some women do go to the tailor, also known as the plastic surgeon, to have the sags tucked.)

Medical folks are divided on how much blame to apportion to gravity and how much to assign to declining levels of estrogen. Some scientists claim that skin changes are just part of aging, but others feel that low levels of estrogen during the years leading up to and after menopause hasten a lot of these changes in your skin.

The hormone-imbalance crowd points out that estrogen helps bring moisture to body tissue. Menopause causes lower levels of *estradiol* (the active kind of estrogen), which causes tissues and mucus membranes all over your body to act strangely. How strangely? Some women develop pimples and dry skin *at the same time.*

But the bottom line here is that during perimenopause and menopause your skin loses its elasticity and tightness — it becomes thinner and saggier. As the fatty layer under your skin thins out over time, it will be easier to see your blood vessels, and you'll bruise more easily. Because your skin is less pliant, it tears more easily than it used to — so you may encounter more minor cuts and scrapes.

Also, the skin-maintenance process slows down as part of the normal aging process in both men and women, so your body doesn't regenerate skin as quickly as it used to — another reason you may bruise and cut more easily and heal more slowly.

Slowing the process down

Whether estrogen treatments are effective in slowing the skin-aging process in menopausal women is still debatable. (Especially because some experts don't believe that shifting hormones have anything to do with skin changes in the first place.) Experts occupy both sides of the fence.

If you want to try an estrogen treatment, skin creams (you can call them *transdermal estradiol therapies* if you're feeling pretentious) seem to be more effective than oral estrogen in preserving skin collagen. But don't get overly optimistic about the results. When you see those smiling, wrinkle-free faces on the estrogen-cream advertisements, you can be sure that it's not the estrogen skin cream that gives those women their smooth skin, big breasts, and girlish figures.

Working on wrinkles

Nothing prevents wrinkles like staying out of the sun. But if the damage has already been done, you can check out products that claim to retard the wrinkling process:

- **Retinoid creams:** These products often make use of the terms *retinoic acid, tretinoin,* and the trademark *Retin-A.* The U.S. Food and Drug Administration wants you to know that retinal skin products are not regulated. That means there's no guarantee about the amount of active ingredients in the product. Retinoids are vitamin-A acids. They work by smoothing out skin pigmentation (color), reducing brown spots and wrinkles, and giving skin a rosy appearance. Usually, several months of use are necessary before you notice any improvement.

  Some people think that, if retinoids are just vitamin A in disguise, they can simply take mega doses of vitamin A to improve their skin. Well, it turns out that vitamin A is toxic in high doses, so it can prove harmful to your health.

- **Alpha-hydroxy creams:** Alpha-hydroxy acids work like a skin peel. They help remove surface skin cells. After these skin cells are removed, your skin looks rosier and smoother. Some advertisers claim that alpha hydroxy helps your skin produce collagen and elastin. If this were true, alpha hydroxy would actually improve the layers under the skin (filling the wrinkles in from the inside out). Unfortunately, these hydroxy creams actually work from the outside in, removing old skin cells and giving your face a glow. Some of the side effects of alpha hydroxy include burning, itching, and general skin pain. Newer products that contain beta-hydroxy acids incorporate a mild aspirin-like substance into the product, which is supposed to eliminate skin irritation.

- **Botox:** Here's one of the newer wrinkle killers. Wrinkles are caused by contraction of facial muscles (as we discuss in the "Making the skin and hormone connection" section of this chapter). Botox, a purified form of the botulism toxin, is injected into the facial muscles. It temporarily removes the wrinkle because the toxin temporarily paralyzes or weakens the affected muscles. When the muscles relax, the wrinkle disappears. Botox treatments usually last for several months before the paralysis wears off and the wrinkle returns.

Shining a light on the sun's dangers

The sun is public enemy number one for the skin. Sun exposure can cause wrinkles when you're in your twenties or early thirties, and it can cause your skin to become leathery and unevenly colored years before perimenopause.

Reining in UV rays

The sun's *ultraviolet rays* (UV) inflict the greatest harm on your skin. UV rays from the sun destroy collagen fibers. Remember, the collagen fibers hold the skin tight and keep it from sagging and wrinkling. The skin has a normal maintenance process in which old skin is sloughed off and new skin is rebuilt. UV radiation messes up this process so that the collagen fibers become disorganized and form "solar scars." Just 5 to 15 minutes of sunbathing for fair- to moderate-skinned people can trash the skin-maintenance process for a week. UV radiation from the sun also causes a buildup of a substance that causes the skin to stretch (*abnormal elastin*).

Caring about skin cancer

Along with lesser problems, UV radiation can cause skin cancer — a serious side effect of too much sun. Skin cancer can show up years after long-term exposure to the sun.

By the time you're menopausal, your risk of skin cancer is higher because you've been exposed to UV radiation for quite a few years. *Malignant melanoma* is a rather rare but deadly form of skin cancer. It's most commonly diagnosed in folks in their early fifties.

When you're in the sun for too long, the sun's UV radiation penetrates your skin and gets down into the DNA inside the skin cells. It zaps and damages the DNA — serious stuff because cell reproduction is based on DNA. Any mistakes in the DNA can have serious ramifications down the line. Sometimes, genetic mutations produce cancerous skin tumors. UV rays also suppress the skin's immune system, leaving your skin susceptible to cancer cells.

Preventing premature skin aging

If you worry about the appearance of your skin, you're probably wondering how you can combat the skin changes that accompany the aging process and menopause. Well, here you go. These are a few ways to keep your skin looking youthful and firm for as long as you can:

✔ **Don't smoke:** On average, smokers have thinner skin and more wrinkles than non-smokers. A heavy smoker is five times more likely to have a wrinkled face than a non-smoker of the same age. A 40-year-old, heavy smoker has the face of a non-smoking 60-year-old in terms of wrinkles.

✔ **Avoid exposure to the sun:** Exposure to ultraviolet radiation accounts for 90 percent of the symptoms of premature skin aging. It's also the most significant cause of skin cancers.

Sniffing Out Nasal Changes

In mid-life, sinus problems hit some women who never had them before. Lower levels of estrogen dry out the mucous membranes in the sinus cavities and nasal passages. "Dry out?" you may be thinking, "But my head feels *stuffy*.

Where's the sense in that?" Here's the deal: Your mucous membranes are supposed to clean out foreign particles from your sinuses and nose. When the membranes are dry, they can't do their job, so your sinuses and nose become inflamed and you develop a case of *chronic rhinitis*. Most folks refer to this condition by a much more scientific name — runny nose.

How do you fix these problems caused by dryness? Instead of using antihistamines or decongestants, which dry you up further, use a saline (salt) nasal spray to moisten mucous tissues and help them work more effectively. Steam baths and hormone therapy also can help relieve the dryness.

Handling Hairy Issues

Gray hair has nothing to do with menopause, except that both tend to occur in women over 40. But menopause does bring about changes in hair patterns in ways you may never have imagined, including losing hair on your head and gaining it on your face.

Here's why hair loss is more likely to happen after menopause: Hair follicles are receptive to hormones. Female hormone (estrogen) levels decrease faster than male hormone (androgen) levels, so where you once had very high levels of active estrogen and very low levels of androgen, you now have low levels of androgen but much lower levels of active estrogen. These lower levels of estrogen aren't enough to block the affect of the androgen.

About one-third of women between the ages of 40 and 80 find their hair thinning all over their scalp but more so on the crown of the head. This is called *female pattern baldness*. The amount of hair loss varies from woman to woman.

Some women have had success using minoxidil, the same treatment recommended for balding men. This medication is better at preserving hair than retrieving what was lost, so if you're going to try it, seek help quickly.

The hormonal imbalance may also cause you to grow a few hairs on your chin or other spots on your face. Hormone therapy helps restore some of the balance between hormones in your body, thus helping to preserve your hair (on your head) and protect your chin from hair growth.

Chapter 8

Menopause and Your Sex Life

*F*riends of my parents were discussing a merry widow who was once again dating and asked, "Why would anyone want to have sex at that age?" And when the same merry widow brags, "Sex is even better after menopause," her more persnickety friends scoff, "Any sex is better than what she was getting." Some folks may interpret the merry old widow as putting too positive of a spin on the change, but rest assured that you don't have to give up sex after sixty. In fact, you may enjoy the experience more than you did when you were concerned about getting pregnant, having the kids burst in at any moment, or finding satisfaction in a quickie when your partner wasn't really in the mood but indulged you anyway.

You may decide that you finally want to use those organs just at a time when they're preparing for retirement. Or you may discover that your organs are still willing, but your hormones are not. If only teenagers had the hormones of a 40-year-old, we'd have far fewer teenage pregnancies! Getting pregnant at 40 isn't impossible, but sometimes, it's not as spontaneous as it can be for women in their twenties.

There's no question that sex changes after menopause — your hormonal changes cause changes in your private parts as well as your emotional parts. But those changes don't mean you need to eliminate sex from your life, and this chapter tells you why. We cover all the issues pertaining to sex for enjoyment and sex for reproduction as you approach, enter, and pass menopause.

Looking at Menopause and Your Libido

Menopause opens a new chapter in your life, so it's no surprise that the sexual you changes as well. In many cases, the changes are for the better. Even though having sex during a menstrual cycle is by no means wrong, most women and their partners refrain from sex for those days. Now that those menstrual periods have hit the road, you have more opportunities for sex. And remember how you always seemed to get your period when you were on vacation, no matter how well you planned? Now you can play around until your heart's content without a visit from "your friend." The crankiness, cramps, and headaches that ebbed and flowed with your menstrual cycle now level out into a kinder and gentler expression of you.

Libido declines with age. That's a fact. Most scientific studies have found that little change in sexual activity occurs between the ages of 45 and 55. But, between 55 and 65, sexual activity slows.

And, though women in their sixties don't engage in sex as often as they did in their younger years, no change occurs in the frequency of orgasm or the level of sexual enjoyment. So, you may not do it as often, but sex is just as satisfying. (An interesting note: Research shows that activity with sexual partners often slows down long before women discontinue masturbating.)

The fluctuating hormones that characterize menopause and perimenopause definitely have an effect on your sex drive. Be prepared for a gradual increase — or a gradual decrease — in your libido. Of course, you may not be aware of any change at all, but most menopausal women experience at least brief periods of higher- or lower-than-usual sex drive.

Letting your feelings be your guide

When it comes down to it, no one knows your body better than you, so pay attention to it. Because every woman experiences menopause a little differently, your medical advisor may not be familiar with your specific symptoms. Learn to trust yourself.

This advice goes double for changes in your *libido* (desire to have sex). Many doctors ignore sexual issues when treating perimenopausal and menopausal women. So, it's important that *you* bring up the issue if your doctor doesn't.

Here are some helpful hints for talking to your doctor:

✔ Doctors have heard everything; don't feel embarrassed about your questions or concerns. If you don't feel comfortable discussing these topics with your doctor, maybe it's time to find one who's more engaging.

✔ Raise your questions early in the appointment. Take a moment right after the "Hi, how are you doing today" part to raise the issue by saying something like, ". . . and doctor there's another problem that we need to solve before I leave today." Don't wait until you're walking out the door to ask your questions.

✔ Keep a diary of any pain, discomfort, or discharge you experience. Track things like how long it lasts, what activity may have caused the problem, and the level of pain you felt.

✔ Sexual responsiveness is a natural process, not a right reserved for special people. If you're experiencing troublesome changes in your sexual desire after menopause, be direct with your doctor. The problem may be hormonal (low testosterone levels), or there may be other medical reasons for the change.

There are many ways to fix this. If your health checks out, you may want to consult a sex therapist (like Dr. Ruth Westheimer). A sex therapist can help you if your problems are behavioral or psychological in nature.

Turning up the heat

More than half of all menopausal women maintain the same level of sexual interest after menopause as before. In fact, you may feel less inhibited when the possibility of pregnancy no longer looms over the bed. Now that you can safely put away some of the contraceptive devices, you're more free to express yourself sexually. Many women report feeling greater sexual creativity and freedom after the change. And many women who experienced a midlife divorce find that sex with their new partner (after menopause) is better than ever.

The famous sex research team of Masters and Johnson proved to the world that sexual *appetite* is not tied to estrogen levels (although you may need a little lubricant to make sex comfortable after estrogen declines). It's really the *androgens* (male sex hormones like testosterone) produced by your ovaries throughout your life that keep your sex drive running. Even after menopause (when your ovaries have gotten out of the estradiol- and progesterone-production game), your ovaries keep on producing androgens.

If you have sex with more than one partner during or after menopause, you still need to practice safe sex to avoid picking up a sexually transmitted disease or AIDS.

Even though men don't go through menopause, their testosterone levels gradually decline after forty. The physiological changes don't happen overnight. Over time, men will notice that it takes longer for them to get an erection and that they aren't aroused as easily, which may be good news for a woman who enjoys foreplay. Women whose partners suffer premature ejaculation can rejoice. That problem goes away and men gain lasting power as they age.

Even if you're having fewer periods (or perhaps you haven't had one in months), don't give up your birth control until you've been without periods for a full year. During perimenopause, your hormone levels and the chance of ovulation are wildly unpredictable. It's unlikely, but you could just have a hormonally hot month and wind up pregnant — everyone knows at least one "change of life" baby.

Dealing with a lowered libido

A healthy self-image and adult lifestyle generally include satisfying and safe sexual activity. Yet many women are frustrated by declining desire for sex during and after menopause. A vital sex life is important to both you and your partner. Understanding the biology behind a declining libido can help bring about a solution.

Your sex drive can decline sooner than you'd like for several reasons. Some are mental or emotional — if your self-esteem declines because of changes in your life or in your body, you may have to address that issue before you can find your old libido. Some of the reasons are physical — painful sex is nothing to look forward to. And some are hormonal — your hormones are changing, and if you'd like to maintain your sex drive, your hormones must be balanced.

Communicating with your doctor and your partner is critical in overcoming decreased libido.

Adjusting your attitude

It's hard to feel amorous when you're depressed. Menopause, in itself, doesn't make you depressed, but think about the types of things happening during these years:

- Kids leaving home
- Parents aging and needing closer attention
- You or your spouse retiring

Add to these challenges the everyday issues of maintaining a happy relationship and just coping in a fast-paced world. Now, the one thing that used to be reliable, your body, is also changing at a faster pace than it has in quite some time. Is it any wonder that sex is the last thing on your mind?

But if the lack of physical spark bothers you, you need to get rid of the emotional stressors before you can expect your libido to kick in. It may just take allocating more time to yourself. Take some time to get an exercise program off the ground. Walking regularly by yourself or with a friend can do plenty to reduce stress. Talk with friends, a therapist, your hairdresser, or minister about your challenges. Also, remember to bring up your anxiety or depression when you talk to your internist or gynecologist.

Making sure that sex isn't a hurtin' thing

Hormonal changes can cause the vaginal lining to become thinner, more fragile, and more susceptible to tearing *and* produce less lubrication. You're more delicate down there — a bit more tender. Vaginal connective tissue also become less pliant, and nerve endings become more sensitive.

The result of this biological shuffle is that intercourse may become painful. Sexual activity that used to deliver great pleasure can now cause pain instead. The thought of the discomfort may make you want to get a headache

It's not the estrogen!

Many reports and books make a huge deal about the fact that no scientific evidence links changes in estrogen levels to a declining libido. These publications then make the leap to erroneously conclude that hormones have nothing to do with libido. Although the estrogen, itself, may not play the deciding role in libido regulation, the *balance* between estrogen and testosterone likely makes a difference.

This subject is a bit controversial so we want to give you both sides of the argument. On one side are scientists who conclude that supplementing your testosterone during menopause increases your libido. On the other side are the lab coats who believe that the science doesn't exist to show that prescribing testosterone is either safe or effective for women who complain of low libido.

Testosterone is produced naturally by women's ovaries and has a very positive impact on your libido, mood, vitality, sense of well-being, bone, and muscle. But, even before menopause, your body slows down its production of testosterone. After menopause, you produce about half as much testosterone as you produced during your reproductive years. So it's not unusual for your libido to decline if your testosterone levels are too low.

You don't want to have too much testosterone either — it can promote breast and liver cancer. Plus, too much testosterone relative to estrogen can unleash the effects of testosterone that estrogen had been keeping under control, such as facial hair, increased libido, redistribution of body fat (it moves to the middle of your body), and acne.

Some doctors shy away from prescribing testosterone as part of hormone therapy (HT) because they're afraid of upsetting the estrogen/testosterone balance and causing unpleasant side effects. The trick, whether you're taking HT with testosterone or not, is to keep testosterone levels high enough to avoid one set of side effects (including low libido) and in balance with the other hormones to avoid another set of side effects (facial hair or acne, for example).

Those folks in the scientific and medical communities who view testosterone as a worthy treatment for libido problems believe that the bad side effects felt by some women are caused by excessively high dosages of testosterone. Proponents of testosterone use suggest using very low dosages and maintaining a balance between the levels of testosterone and estrogen.

or clean out your sock drawer when your partner makes amorous advances, but all is not lost. You can alleviate painful intercourse in a variety of ways:

- ✔ **Maintain an active sex life.** Regular sexual activity keeps blood circulating in your vulva and slows the drying process. So maintaining an active sex life helps postpone or altogether avoid the pain associated with dry vaginal tissues.

- ✔ **Talk to your partner about the more sensitive you.** Most men aren't aware that hormonal changes trigger changes in your vulva and vagina. Explain to your partner that the two of you need to figure out new bedroom strategies that can be mutually satisfying.

- ✔ **Use a lubricant during intercourse to help keep things moving.** Lubricants can afford hours of interpersonal pleasure. Some women and their partners make lubricant application a part of foreplay. Water-based lubricants, such as Astroglide, are healthier for vaginal linings.

Sometimes women experience regular discomfort due to vaginal dryness — not just during sex. If you're one of them, you can use other types of lubricants on a regular basis to relieve this irritation. (See the product literature for recommended dosage, and check out Chapter 6 on tips for dealing with vaginal dryness.)

Don't use estrogen cream as a sexual lubricant. The estrogen cream can be absorbed by your partner and cause problems. At least one case of breast cancer has been reported in a man because his wife used vaginal estrogen cream as a lubricant. It's important to read the instructions!

Talking Turkey about Testosterone

Don't forget that men, as well as women, experience declining libido as they age! If you're noticing changes in your sexual relationship, remember that your partner's hormones are changing too. Men produce much more testosterone than women, but when they reach 40, their testosterone levels begin declining. However, most men don't notice an appreciable change in their libido for about another 10 years. Around the age of 50 or so, the drop in testosterone causes men to stop having *psychogenic erections* (erections from just thinking about sex), and men who could have an erection at the drop of a hat find that it's a bit harder (no pun intended) to get things moving.

So, if you're worried because your partner isn't pursuing you like he used to, your menopause may not be at the heart of the matter. Your partner may be going through hormonal changes of his own, even though his change isn't as dramatic as yours.

Keeping Sex Sexy

If you've noticed some changes in your sexual relationship, work with your partner to make things better. Your relationship can evolve to a new level of meaning and pleasure.

First, you need to communicate with your partner and take stock of the situation. Is it a libido thing for you? Is it a libido thing for him? Is it technique? Is it timing? You need to find out what's going on.

As you and your partner get older and both your testosterone levels decline, it's time to spend more time on foreplay. You may both need more stimulation before intercourse. And you may need to incorporate lubricants into your foreplay if you have vaginal dryness.

You may also have to incorporate different techniques to provide enough stimulation for your man to get an erection — you may have to work a little magic to get his penis into position at this stage of his life. Hand stimulation or oral sex may be what it takes to get him started. You can also turn to books and counselors — two good sources of information on sexual techniques and other sexual matters for mature adults. You can find a sex therapist on the Internet at `www.psychology.com/therapy`.

Although we baby-boomers come from the "sex, booze, and drugs" generation, these words no longer work together. Take a look at some of the things that can douse your flame:

- **Alcohol:** One drink may make you feel relaxed and less inhibited, but several drinks can put a damper on your libido, your ability to become aroused, your performance, and your ability to reach orgasm.

- **Prescription drugs:** Serotonin boosters, antidepressants, blood pressure pills, sleeping pills, and many other drugs frequently prescribed for women over 50 can take a toll on your libido. Let your gynecologist and internist know what medications you take when you discuss your libido and sexual performance. Alternative medications may be available that can alleviate some of the negative side effects.

- **Tobacco products:** The nicotine in cigarettes and other tobacco products constricts the blood vessels making it more difficult for blood to rush to your private parts. It's harder to get aroused and harder still to experience a satisfactory conclusion.

Diabetes and other medical problems also cause loss of sexual desire and performance problems. Be sure to consult with your doctor about changes in your libido because they can result from other medical conditions.

To Fertility and Beyond

The hormone dance that ends in menopause actually begins years before you stop having periods. Most women don't know what time the ball begins and are shocked when they have trouble getting pregnant in their thirties.

In fact, according to a recent study, a woman's fertility begins to decline in her late twenties, rather than her thirties as previously thought. Researchers found that even women in their early- to mid-twenties have only a fifty-fifty chance of becoming pregnant each cycle even if they have intercourse during the peak time for conception. In your late twenties to early thirties, the chance drops to 40 percent each cycle, and by the late thirties it's less than a 30 percent chance. Figure 8-1 shows the odds per cycle

By the way, that study also finds that men's fertility also begins to decline sooner than expected. Men begin to lose their fertility in their thirties rather than in the forties as was once thought. So if you're in your late thirties and your partner is five years older than you are, your chances of becoming pregnant in any given cycle could drop to 20 percent.

This just means that you have to try for more cycles to get pregnant. It doesn't mean that you won't conceive if you're in your late thirties; it just means that it may take a few months longer, especially if your partner is older than you are.

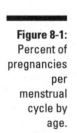

Figure 8-1:
Percent of pregnancies per menstrual cycle by age.

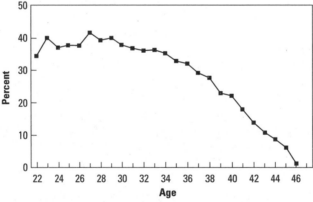

Many women who put off motherhood until their late thirties need a little help to get pregnant. Fertility treatment programs that help women get pregnant are multiplying like bunnies across the United States. Read on to discover what fertility treatment is all about.

Evaluating whether it's too late to start a family

You may have had the same experience that we had when we were teenagers: Parents, teachers, and even friends had us believing that practically all you had to do to get pregnant was to jump in a swimming pool with a boy. Okay, that's a slight exaggeration, but generally, getting pregnant is easier when you're in your teens than when you're in your thirties.

The word medical folks use to describe women who have trouble getting pregnant is *infertile*. We don't really like that word because it makes it sound like a woman is a patch of windswept desert. Plus, with treatment, many "infertile" women become pregnant. *Infertility* is usually defined as the inability to get pregnant after trying for one year.

Getting a head start on the pregnancy thing

To optimize your chances of getting pregnant, here are some things you can work on before you see a doctor:

- Be sure your diet is healthy (five fruits and vegetables each day).
- Exercise regularly.
- Plan your sexual activities to optimize your chances of getting pregnant. Have intercourse several times during your ovulation cycle (see the "Figuring out when you're fertile" sidebar in this chapter).
- Rid your life of as much stress as you can. Take a vacation, get plenty of rest, and stay on an even keel emotionally.

Knowing when you're fertile, Myrtle

You're most fertile right before and during ovulation. Some women can tell when they ovulate because they feel a dull pain in the area of their ovary. But this is a rare talent, and most women need to employ a trick or two. The simplest and cheapest test: Take your temperature (we turn your attention to the "Figuring out when you're fertile" sidebar in this chapter). Using temperature charts is an accurate ovulation test, but you have to stick with it and take your temperature everyday beginning on the first day of your period. Also, you only find out that you've ovulated after the fact. Figure 8-2 shows a sample ovulation chart.

If you need to know if you're ovulating right away and you haven't been taking your temperature, test kits are available in grocery stores and pharmacies. You can buy ovulation test kits over the counter, and they're easy to use.

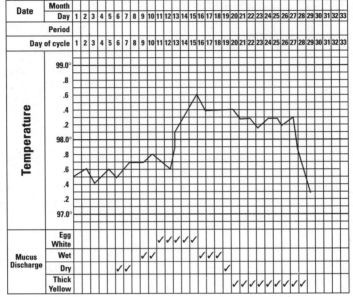

Figure 8-2:
One
woman's
record of
her fertility
cycle.

When you ovulate, the *follicle* (the little sac that holds the egg) in your ovary releases an egg, and the egg begins a little journey down the fallopian tube and into the uterus. The egg lives for anywhere between 6 and 24 hours after ovulation. Because the sperm can live for two to seven days inside a woman (if she has good, fertile mucus), having sex just prior to and during ovulation is the best way to go. Men can make about 50,000 sperm a minute, but it just takes one to make a baby.

Tracing the yin and yang of conception

Many things have to happen correctly to make a baby:

- ✔ Your ovaries must produce follicles.

- ✔ The follicles have to grow big enough to release an egg.

- ✔ Your hormones have to be just right for the egg to be released and survive the journey.

- ✔ Your fallopian tubes must be unobstructed so that the egg can swim all the way through to the uterus to meet some nice sperm.

- ✔ Your hormones must create the right type of environment for the egg to get fertilized and comfortably nestled into the lining of the uterus.

Out of whack hormones (and that's the technical term — not!) are to blame for most of the infertility problems perimenopausal women face.

Facing up to potential problems

The previous section tells you everything that needs to go right in order for a woman to get pregnant. Now check out some of the more common things that go wrong during attempts to conceive and what can be done about these problems:

- ✔ **Problem:** Your ovaries aren't producing follicles or the follicles never get big enough to produce an egg because your hormones are out of balance.

  Medical tests: Your doctor will likely perform a series of tests. First, he or she will do blood tests at several points throughout your cycle to determine if your hormones are at the right levels to produce follicles, ovulate, and provide safe harbor for a fertilized egg in your uterus. If all is well with your hormones, your doctor may take a peak at your ovaries using a sonogram (ultrasound) at about the midway point of your cycle to see if you're making healthy follicles and to see if your follicles are growing to a healthy size. You can also check your progesterone on Day 21 to see if ovulation occurred.

  Solutions: Your doctor may have you take fertility medications to help you produce more follicles.

- ✔ **Problem:** After the egg is released, your fallopian tube may be obstructed so the egg can't make it to the uterus.

  Medical tests: A *laparoscopy* to look at your tubes to see if they're obstructed and examine other organs to see if they are diseased. Another common test is called a *hysterosalpingogram.* A dye is injected and an x-ray is taken of the fallopian tubes and uterus to see if the tubes are open and the uterus is in good shape.

  Solutions: Sometimes the test finds evidence of endometriosis, which can be treated with surgery or medication.

- ✔ **Problem:** The endometrium (lining of the uterus) may not get thick enough for the fertilized egg to latch onto and snuggle in.

  Medical test: *Endometrial biopsy* to rule out a hormonal deficiency. You may be low on progesterone so your endometrium doesn't get thick enough for a fertilized egg to nestle in.

  Solution: Your doctor may put you on a hormone regimen of progesterone after ovulation.

If you and your partner seek professional help with fertility, both of you will be tested and treatment will depend on those initial tests. A normal series of semen analyses will prompt a workup for you; an abnormal series will prompt a workup for him.

Figuring out when you're fertile

There are three good ways to figure out when you're fertile, and we tell you about all three here.

Basal body temperature (BBT) method

Recording your *basal body temperature* (BBT) is a very easy and accurate way to find out when you're ovulating. It works on the principle that your body temperature rises (anywhere from 0.6 to 1.0 degrees Fahrenheit) when you produce higher levels of progesterone. Your body begins to produce more progesterone as you ovulate, and continues to produce progesterone to prepare your uterus for an embryo, so after ovulation, your body temperature continues to rise for a few days. If you're not pregnant, your temperature drops back down.

Here's how you do it:

1. Take your temperature orally every morning for several months just after you wake up (before you eat, drink, or do anything). Use a special ovulation thermometer that can distinguish even very small temperature changes — in tenths of a degree — or a digital thermometer that registers by tenths. Leave the thermometer in place for a full 5 minutes. **Important:** Shake down the thermometer immediately after you record the temperature; do not wait until the next morning because even the activity of shaking down the thermometer can raise your basal temperature.

2. Record your temperature on a chart or graph every day. Ovulation usually causes your BBT to increase by 0.6°F to 1.0°F and to remain high for over a week. Ovulation occurs sometime between the day when your temperature begins to rise and the day it reaches its highest point.

You're fertile during the three days of higher temperature. Sperm can live for 48 to 72 hours.

Continue to record your temperature for at least three months using a new chart for each menstrual cycle. (See the chart in Figure 8-2 to find out what this should look like.) This way you'll be able to tell if you're ovulating and the cycle day upon which you typically start ovulating, and you'll get to know your body's pattern. It's a good idea to continue charting your BBT as long as you're trying to get pregnant.

Cervical mucus method (Billings method)

Another test involves keeping tabs on your vaginal mucus, which changes color, texture, and quantity throughout your cycle. This is a very accurate method, but it takes some practice to recognize the changes.

Here's how you do it:

1. Every day, insert your finger into your vagina. Your finger should come out damp with mucus. (Don't test after intercourse because it will be hard to distinguish mucus from semen.) Check out the amount, color, and thickness (or thinness) of the mucus.

2. Test the "stretchiness" of the mucus by touching your thumb to the finger you inserted and slowly spreading your finger and thumb; note how long the strand of mucus becomes before it breaks.

If you happen to have a microscope handy, you can spread some mucus on a thin piece of glass and let it dry, then look at it under a microscope to see whether it dried in a fernlike pattern.

3. Now, write down all of your assessments on a calendar. Here's what you should notice:

✔ After your period, your mucus tends to be very scant, cloudy, whitish to yellow, and slightly sticky.

✔ Just before ovulation, the mucus increases in amount, becomes clear and slippery, stretches more than 1 inch before it breaks, and dries in a fernlike pattern.

The time for sexual action, if you want to become pregnant, begins the day you notice your cervical mucus becoming clear and stretchable until the day it becomes cloudy and sticky.

Combined method

If you're not a scientist, evaluating your cervical mucus can be challenging. To give you a heads up on what to look for in your mucus, you may want to also keep track of your BBT so that you'll know approximately where you are in your cycle when you're studying your bodily fluid. Track both the BBT and your mucus observations on a calendar.

See Chapter 2 for more detailed information on what happens during each phase of your menstrual cycle.

Taking a dipstick to your estrogen

When you seek some assistance in your bid to get pregnant, one of the first things fertility doctors do is check to see if you're capable of ovulating. In order to ovulate, you need both the right kind of estrogen and the right amount of this particular form of estrogen in your bloodstream. This form of estrogen is called *estradiol,* and your doctor will take a blood sample to check your estradiol out.

As you approach menopause, your body produces less estradiol but continues to produce estrone. When it comes to producing follicles and ovulating, estradiol is the kind that counts: Without adequate levels of estradiol, your ovaries won't produce an egg. By measuring both types of estrogen, your doctor can see whether you're heading toward menopause or whether you have some other hormonal problems. (See Chapter 2 for more info on the different types of hormones women produce.)

Because your hormone levels fluctuate during perimenopause, you may still have periods, but you may not ovulate each month. Your estradiol levels may be sufficiently high one month and be low another month. Some months are good for getting pregnant and some months are not so good. By measuring your estradiol levels each month, your doctor will be able to see if it's a good month for producing an egg or not.

Messing up the nest with hormones

Sometimes hormonal problems occur after the follicle releases the egg. Normally the follicle pops open to release the egg and then hangs around long enough to produce progesterone (after the follicle releases the egg, the empty sac is called a *corpus luteum*). The corpus luteum eventually disintegrates.

Progesterone production is necessary for thickening the uterine lining and preparing it for the egg. If the follicle doesn't produce enough progesterone, problems arise that can put an end to conception. If the lining isn't ready, the fertilized egg won't nestle into the endometrium properly.

Progesterone production slows down during perimenopause and menopause, so you may have problems making a home for a fertilized egg.

Having periods doesn't mean you're fertile

Even for women in their prime baby-conceiving years, the planets need to be aligned to get pregnant. But as you move into your perimenopausal years, some months you ovulate, and some months you don't. As time goes by, you experience more and more cycles in which you don't ovulate.

You may have a period even if you don't ovulate.

Getting pregnant outside the bedroom

Couples have trouble getting pregnant for many reasons. The reasons described in this chapter are some of the more common problems triggered by hormonal imbalances in perimenopausal women. If you're having trouble getting pregnant after 30, seek help from your gynecologist or a fertility specialist.

A full coverage of fertility treatments would take another complete book, so we just hit some of the highlights. Your gynecologist should be able to refer you to a fertility treatment clinic. And, if you're past your prime in terms of the fertility game, today's fertility clinics have a host of conception alternatives outside the bedroom. Fertility is a seven-days-a-week issue. Fertility clinics will schedule your visits according to your needs, even if you need a procedure on Thanksgiving!

So what are the chances of becoming pregnant? Obviously your chances of becoming pregnant depend on your individual circumstances but some fertility clinics have conception rates as high as 50 percent, meaning that half of their patients are successful at conceiving under their care.

If you have ethical or religious concerns about artificial reproductive therapy, these options may not be right for you.

Here are some of the fertility techniques in use today:

AI: Artificial insemination

If the reproduction problems you're experiencing relate to the sperm, you may want to consider artificial insemination. In artificial insemination, a doctor places semen into your uterus or vaginal canal using a tiny tube. Think of this procedure as a head start for the backstroke-challenged sperm.

Mother's little helper: In vitro fertilization

If you're having problems conceiving, another alternative is *in vitro* fertilization. In this procedure, doctors give the woman medication to stimulate her ovaries to produce several eggs. This medicine stimulates her ovaries to produce three to ten eggs in a cycle (you normally produce only one or two per cycle). When the eggs are mature, the physician suctions the eggs out of the ovaries and puts them in a lab dish. Your partner will "make a specimen" to fertilize the eggs. (It's best if the ejaculate is fresh, but you can use frozen sperm or even sperm from a donor.) The doctor takes the sperm, mixes it with the eggs, and tucks the dish containing the sperm and eggs into an incubator. After a few days, the doctor checks the dish to see if any of the eggs were fertilized. With luck, one or more have been fertilized and the doctor replants the embryos into the woman's body. Then the woman waits to see if the embryos latch onto the lining of the uterus, making her pregnant.

In vitro fertilization has no guarantees. The procedure is expensive and presents risks to the health of the patient. The medication may raise the risk of cancer, and your ovaries may be overstimulated into producing a whole lot of follicles, which can be uncomfortable. Finally, you may have great success in producing lots of eggs and producing multiple embryos. The risks to the lives and health of the mom and babies go up astronomically when more than two or three babies are in the womb. But in vitro fertilization is an alternative to be considered by women who have had trouble conceiving.

Taking the good with the bad

There's good news, and there's bad news when the subject at hand is conception and the older woman. Because we don't want you walking away from this chapter on a down note, we start off this section with a few gloomy stats and then turn our attention to the good stuff.

Around the time women hit the 35-to-38 mark (some experts say as early as 30), their fertility gradually declines, and it drops precipitously at 40. Unfortunately, around this time, a woman's risk of spontaneous miscarriage begins to rise. By age 45, women have a fifty-fifty chance of suffering a spontaneous miscarriage if they conceive. Also, by the time women reach 45, the risk of chromosomal abnormalities in the baby increases to 1 chance in 40. In other words, for every 40 babies conceived by women 45 or older, one baby has a chromosomal abnormality such as Down syndrome or spina bifida.

But there are also advantages to becoming a mom for the first time after 40. For example, the perimenopausal symptom of interrupted sleep means that you'll probably already be awake when the baby cries. You and the newborn will be on the same wavelength, and you'll have someone to talk to when you wake up.

Women who have waited to have families are typically better prepared for the sacrifices they need to make to nurture children. Both of us waited to start our families and have found that we're in much better positions to devote our time and attention to our children than we would have been in our twenties. Establishing careers, entertaining friends, travel, and other interests often preoccupy life during your twenties and thirties. Now you may be more willing to make time to raise a family.

Chapter 9

Mental and Emotional Issues

. . . .

In This Chapter

▶ Remembering to read this chapter

▶ Recognizing emotional changes during menopause

▶ Getting a handle on your headaches

▶ Connecting hormones to mental and emotional stress

. . . .

*M*any of us have "senior moments" even before menopause. You know —
those times when you forget how to spell simple words like *apple*. (Is it
le or *el?*) Or you're about to introduce a friend you've known for years and her
name suddenly escapes you. Or maybe you find yourself spending more time
thinking about the hereafter — as in, "What am I here after?"

You're not alone. Many women experience these mental lapses during perimenopause or menopause. Some women even experience this type of forgetfulness long before menopause — during their menstrual cycle when
estrogen levels are at their lowest. Estrogen plays a major role in memory
and emotional functions.

Some perimenopausal and menopausal women also fall prey to emotional
slumps. Fluctuating hormone levels prompt some emotional moments
(remember being a moody adolescent?); others can come as a reaction to the
symptoms you're dealing with or the stage of life you're in.

Thank goodness not all women experience mental and emotional problems
during perimenopause or menopause. Like PMS (premenstrual syndrome),
these symptoms are more severe in some women than others. Some women
just seem to be more sensitive to hormonal changes. In fact, if you had
memory lapses and heightened emotions in connection with your menstrual
cycle in the past, they may be part of your perimenopausal and menopausal
experience too.

In this chapter, we cover some of the symptoms you may be experiencing, how they're related to your hormones, and how you can tell if a symptom is hormonal or psychological.

Understanding the Mental and Emotional Stresses of Menopause

Fortunately, with 40 or 50 years of emotional experience behind you, you're quite prepared to cope with the challenges life throws your way. Midlife changes present you with openings — and you can view openings either as voids or opportunities for new experiences.

If emotional issues or mental lapses bother you during these years, visit your medical advisor. Life events may trigger temporary mental or emotional issues, but there's a difference between a temporary mental state and a debilitating condition. If your emotional state severely interferes with your daily life for a prolonged period of time, visit a therapist or counselor.

Many physical conditions, not just menopause, can lead to mental and emotional problems — but menopause is certainly one of these conditions.

The medical establishment didn't recognize hot flashes as an actual physical condition (as opposed to whining) until the late 1970s, so you may not be surprised to hear that doctors sometimes forget to take hormones into consideration when women experience mental or emotional symptoms. Even if you ask, "Do you think it could be related to menopause?" your doctor may say, "You're too young to be going into menopause," or "It can't be menopause, you're still having periods."

Sometimes you, the patient, must take that bull by the horns (or by the hormones), and educate your medical advisor: The symptoms caused by estrogen fluctuations are at least as common in perimenopause as they are during menopause itself. You may have to insist on a test to check your hormone levels. And if you meet resistance, ask your friends for the name of a more receptive doctor.

You have estrogen receptors all over your brain, particularly in areas associated with memory and mood, because your brain needs estrogen to function properly. So, a dip in your estrogen levels can affect your mental and emotional health.

You may actually experience some of the mental/emotional symptoms associated with menopause during your regular menstrual cycle. Hormone levels shift throughout the menstrual cycle, so you have a few low-estrogen days just before starting your period (see Chapter 2 for details on your hormone rhythms).

You may be familiar with those three little letters — PMS (premenstrual syndrome). Unfortunately, PMS was just an appetizer for the main course. Memory lapses, fuzzy thinking, depression, anxiety, and mood swings — all those pleasant memories from your youth — can show up at your door for a longer visit during perimenopause and menopause. And no, you can't turn off the lights and pretend that you're not at home like you do when *those* family members show up unannounced.

Separating menopausal symptoms from psychological disorders

When we talk about the mental and emotional changes you may experience during perimenopause and menopause, it's important to distinguish between these symptoms and the psychological disorders of the same name. For example, some women experience periods of depression during menopause. How do you know if you're in trouble or if this is just a symptom you have to deal with?

During perimenopause and menopause, going through bouts of depression isn't unusual. During your younger days, you may have felt moody or blue for a few days each month before your period. But most women in their forties and fifties have to deal with physiological changes (like they did when they were younger) while they're dealing with life-changing events such as their parents aging, the death of a loved one, marital problems, empty nests, retirement, and maybe job loss.

We all feel sad, dejected, or blue now and then. You may become upset when you look in the mirror and see someone who has a few more wrinkles today than last year or someone who still hasn't won the Nobel prize. Or you may be in the midst of profound mourning after the death of a loved one. Such sorrow may last for several months — which is a completely normal response to a deeply-felt emotional loss. The major difference between sad feelings and a true major depression is that sad feelings eventually pass — depression doesn't.

Depression (with a capital D) envelops you as a sort of psychic cloud, numbing you with thoughts that the bleak outlook will never change. A psychological disorder like depression interferes with sleep, appetite, sexual interest, self-image, and attitude. Herein lies the problem of determining whether you're experiencing depression or perimenopausal/menopausal symptoms — the hormonal changes also interfere with your sleep, mood, and libido. But when you don't snap out of your dark mood — the cloud doesn't lift after weeks, months, or years — you move into the category of psychological disorder.

The mental and emotional changes that you experience because of hormonal changes shouldn't interfere with your daily life — cause damage to friendships or relationships with the folks at work, make it impossible to manage your normal schedule of activities, or prompt you to use alcohol or drugs to help you feel better. If your symptoms do provoke these changes, talk to your doctor, seek out psychological help, or talk to your spiritual advisor.

You typically experience symptoms of menopause over a limited period of time, in episodes that come and go as your hormone levels fluctuate. Although your loved ones may disagree, these symptoms don't completely alter your everyday life. They may make you occasionally unpleasant to be around for a while, but they're not debilitating.

Dealing with the head games

Your memory works because *neurons* (nerve cells) talk to each other via neural connectors. Neurons and neural connectors get damaged over time — that's normal. A decrease in estrogen can also cause problems because estrogen stimulates your brain to build more neural connectors.

The mind games associated with menopause are tricky, and they come on gradually — so gradually that you're not sure whether you've always been this way or if this is something new. You think you're going crazy. Your brain just doesn't seem to be working the way it used to! Some of the symptoms you may experience include

- **Fuzzy thinking:** Having trouble staying focused at work? Do you feel like you're walking around in a fog some days? Many women complain of problems concentrating during perimenopause and menopause. Shortened attention spans also seem to be associated with hormonal change.

- **Headaches:** Some women who experienced migraines during their menstrual cycles lose them after menopause. Other women first begin getting migraines during menopause, or their migraines worsen with menopause.

  More women than men get migraines, and the headaches generally start after puberty, which seems to indicate a connection to female sex hormones. But the connection is strange. Blood vessels constrict with migraines, but estrogen helps dilate blood vessels — making you think that the estrogen in hormone therapy (HT) would help migraines. But some women on HT actually get worse migraines with treatment, while other women get estrogen-withdrawal headaches from a decrease in that hormone. So, medical folks still don't see the connection between estrogen and headaches.

✔ **Memory lapses:** Not everyone experiences memory lapses, but if you do, they can be annoying. Losing your car keys or temporarily forgetting how to spell a simple word is aggravating, but not recognizing your husband or child is another story altogether. Just because you occasionally experience this can't-find-my-pencil type of memory loss doesn't mean that you have Alzheimer's disease or that you're going to develop it.

Finding the pieces

Researchers still don't know all the specifics of how estrogen helps your brain remember, but we do know that estrogen helps build healthy connections between neurons in your brain. Estrogen also facilitates blood flow to the brain by dilating blood vessels and relaxing them (so they don't develop spasms). (See Chapter 5 for more on how estrogen keeps your blood vessels healthy.) Both of these effects of estrogen keep your mind from going to mush.

Because estrogen plays a big part in regulating brain function, you may wonder if women who take HT have fewer mental symptoms than other menopausal women. The answer is yes. A recent study of healthy menopausal women (healthy meaning they showed no signs of dementia) found that those using estrogen had better short-term memory than those not taking estrogen.

Women can show improvement after as little as three weeks of HT. With hormone therapy, women improved verbal memory, mental concentration, reasoning, and motor speed.

Estrogen levels must rise to a certain level to have a positive affect on memory, so make sure a doctor evaluates your estrogen levels through a blood test and changes your dosage of HT if no improvement in memory is observed after treatment begins.

Beating the memory game

The least invasive (and a very effective) way to improve your memory during and after menopause is one that also improves the rest of your health: Subscribe to a balanced diet and exercise regularly. Also remember (no pun intended; well, okay, it was intended) that your brain needs exercise too. Whether you're 5 years old or 50, you need to exercise your brain (we provide some suggestions in the following bullets) to keep those neurons active and improve your memory. Here are some ways to boost your memory:

✔ **Check your thyroid and ovarian hormone levels:** Checking your hormone levels can help determine whether your symptoms are related to menopause or whether you may have a more serious condition.

✔ **Don't smoke:** Among the other undesirable effects of smoking, those gray clouds suffocate the nerve cells as they restrict the amount of oxygen that gets to your brain.

✔ **Exercise your mental muscle:** Do crossword puzzles, read, take a class, or try memorizing poems or recipes. Stimulating your brain helps you build new neural connections.

✔ **Exercise your body:** Walk, swim, or do yoga. We don't care which exercise you choose, just get moving. Brisk aerobic activity three to five times a week for 30 minutes to an hour keeps the oxygen flowing to your brain, which improves your memory and your mood.

✔ **Get enough sleep:** A loss of estrogen can cause disruptions in your sleep. Whether your particular brand of sleep deprivation is due to stress, urinary problems, low levels of estrogen, or your partner's snoring, it can do a number on your memory.

Be careful about using sleeping pills; they interrupt your normal sleep patterns, which in turn, has a negative impact on your memory. You should never use sleeping pills for more than two weeks in a row.

✔ **Limit your alcohol consumption:** Alcohol damages nerve cells in the brain and depletes your body of vitamins necessary for building neural connections. You should limit your alcohol consumption to no more than three drinks each week.

✔ **Take your vitamins:** Certain vitamins help build nerve cells and the neural connectors that you need to remember things (or to just plain think). Some of the more important vitamins include

  • **B vitamins:** This group includes vitamins B1, B2, B6, and B12. You can find vitamin B in meat, enriched flour, and wheat germ.

  • **Folic acid:** Folic acid actually belongs to the family of B vitamins. But, unlike many other B vitamins, this one is found primarily in vegetables rather than flour and meat. Green leafy vegetables, like spinach, collard greens, kale, and broccoli, are rich in folic acid.

  • **Antioxidants:** The antioxidants serve as rust protection for your cells. Oxidation of your cells has a similar effect as oxidation of metal (called rust) — it damages and eventually kills your cells. Antioxidants include vitamins E and C, beta carotene, and selenium.

Take a look at Chapter 18 to find out more about the importance of vitamins during and after menopause. Most women require a multivitamin to get sufficient dosages of these vitamins.

Connecting estrogen and Alzheimer's

When you catch yourself forgetting something, your first thought may be, "Oh my gosh, I have Alzheimer's!" You're referring to the dementia associated with Alzheimer's. *Dementia* is the loss of intellectual abilities such as memory, judgment, and orientation. Alzheimer's is just one of many causes of dementia.

Research into Alzheimer's is in its infancy. Scientists know that the disease damages neurons in the parts of the brain responsible for memory, speech, emotions, and thinking, but they still haven't discovered exactly why this happens.

Estrogen appears to play some role in the disease. Receptors for sex hormones, such as estrogen, progesterone, and testosterone, are located in the parts of the brain that Alzheimer's disease damages. Researchers also know that estrogen stimulates the growth of nerve connections. One study showed that women who were on hormone therapy (HT) were about half as likely to have Alzheimer's as women who weren't on HT. In another study, women with Alzheimer's seemed to improve slightly when put on HT.

Straightening out the commotions with your emotions

As a woman, if you're going to develop depression or an anxiety disorder in your lifetime, it will most likely happen when you're in your late thirties or early forties. A hormonal link between depression and menopause seems to exist. Aside from this fairly obvious coincidence in timing, some physical characteristics of women with depression point to lower levels of estrogen as a factor: Women with depression tend to have lower estrogen levels, and their estrogen levels go up after they pull out of the depression. Also, women with depression have lower bone density than non-depressed women. Low bone density is another common byproduct of low estrogen levels.

Feeling your way through the symptoms

Here are the emotional changes you may notice as you approach menopause:

- ✔ **Anxiety:** You're driving along and all of a sudden you feel panicky. With anxiety, you may experience both emotional and physical symptoms. Emotionally you may be irritable or have trouble focusing. Physically, your heart may start beating like you've just sprinted the 50-yard dash. You wonder if you should drive straight to the hospital. Heart *palpitations* or a racing heart accompanied by butterflies in your stomach are common during perimenopause and menopause.

✔ **Depression:** If you're dealing with interrupted sleep, hot flashes, or memory lapses, avoiding depression altogether is hard. If you experienced depression related to PMS or if you had to deal with postpartum (after-childbirth) depression, you're more likely to experience depression during the change.

✔ **Increased sensitivity:** You may feel that life isn't fair or that everything is your fault, or you may find yourself looking for a fight. Performing at any level that falls short of perfection can cause a negative emotional reaction. Or you may experience crying jags — with or without reason.

✔ **Mood swings:** One minute everything is fine, and the next minute you're sad and gloomy. You may find it difficult dealing with family situations, relationships at home, or professional relationships.

Understanding the physiology and getting relief

When estrogen levels drop, the hormone *serotonin* decreases. Serotonin helps decrease anxiety, so when it drops, you tend to get more anxious. When serotonin drops, it also aggravates adrenalin-inspired irritability and heart palpitations in addition to anxiety. Your doctor may prescribe serotonin-enhancing antidepressants to relieve anxiety during perimenopause and menopause.

Selective serotonin-reuptake inhibitors (SSRIs) have come to the rescue of perimenopausal and menopausal women. SSRIs can balance certain brain chemicals. When these brain chemicals are in proper balance, the symptoms of depression are often relieved.

SSRIs are also used to treat depression triggered by an imbalance between estrogen and progesterone in your body. With estrogen levels lower during perimenopause and menopause, progesterone can temporarily overpower the effects of estrogen and testosterone in your brain. You may feel like crying, or you may feel irritable, grumpy, or downright ugly.

Anxiety and depression can also be treated without medication through acupuncture, biofeedback, yoga, relaxation, herbal remedies, and massage. (See Chapter 16 for more information on alternative therapies.)

Your forties and fifties are a time of change — not only in your body but also in your everyday routines. These lifestyle changes can exacerbate the hormonal dance happening in your body.

Situational stress triggers changes in ovarian function. When the ovaries are hit with stress, such as stress caused the lifestyle changes we discuss in the following sections, hormone production can drop off causing emotional changes. It's a vicious circle: Certain life events cause mood swings, and the mood swings trigger changes in your internal hormones that exaggerate the swing. So life events may start your mental and emotional symptoms, but hormonal changes turn up the volume.

Managing a family

Raising children is always an emotional experience. Everyone knows you're superwoman, but step back and put the whole picture in perspective. You're at midlife, and you're juggling a host of responsibilities: a job, childcare, household chores, a marriage, and maybe an aging parent or in-law. No wonder you're a little scatterbrained and walking around in a fog. You wouldn't change your situation for the world, but caring for a family during menopause can leave you deprived of sleep, irritable, and feeling a bit moody.

Caring for aging parents

Face it, when you hit midlife, your parents may be hitting their golden years. Baby boomers are often called the *sandwich generation* because so many of us find ourselves caring for aging parents while trying to hold down the fort at home with our kids. We often find ourselves parenting 80-year-olds and 4-year-olds at the same time — which is harder? The anxiety of trying to manage multiple households and meet the care needs of those who are closest to us is a very legitimate reason in and of itself for feeling guilty, inadequate, depressed, and irritable. Throw hormonal imbalance into the mix and things get really crazy. It's not just menopause; it's life!

Experiencing the empty nest (Or wishing your nest was empty)

When some women hit menopause, the kids are either leaving home, have recently left home, or *should* have left home. The house seems strangely quiet, the routines you've had for 18 or more years are interrupted, and you feel a simultaneous sense of freedom and loneliness. The world that used to revolve around high-school events comes to a screeching halt, creating a void and an opportunity all at the same time.

Or maybe your kids are just teenagers when you reach menopause. The teenage years can fill a family with turmoil because the house is full of people whose hormones are in flux. After all, a lot of similarities can be drawn between puberty and menopause when it comes to hormonal imbalances and the associated mental/emotional changes.

Retiring, gracefully or not

Whether it's you or your partner, ending a career can be emotionally challenging. Like sending your kids off into the world after high school, the abrupt shift in day-to-day routines that accompanies retirement adds stress to your life. Even if you've been counting down the days until retirement, the change can play some games with your emotions. If you've been used to getting your "that-a-girls" at work, you may find that your self-esteem takes a hit after retirement. How in the world are they able to get along at work without you? With extra time on your hands, you may feel unneeded. Who woulda thought you'd miss being in the center of the action at work?

No matter what your exact situation is, you have plenty of good reasons to be at a heightened emotional stage during midlife. It's not just the hormone thing; it's the everyday world you live in during your forties and fifties.

Part III
Treating the Effects

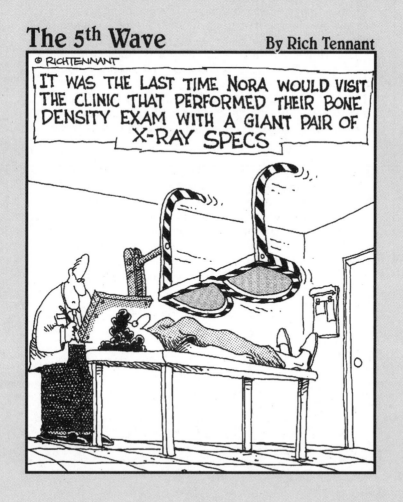

The 5th Wave
By Rich Tennant

IT WAS THE LAST TIME NORA WOULD VISIT THE CLINIC THAT PERFORMED THEIR BONE DENSITY EXAM WITH A GIANT PAIR OF X-RAY SPECS

In this part . . .

*I*f you're like most women, the barrage of newsflashes and special reports on hormone therapy that seem to pop up a few times a year may leave your head spinning. Flash: "Never take hormones." Report: "Never stop taking hormones." Getting a handle on the risks and benefits of hormone therapy can be challenging. In this part, we attempt to demystify the subject, so that you're in a position to make informed decisions (with the assistance of your medical advisor) about whether hormone therapy is right for you.

In the chapters that follow, we present you with the latest information regarding hormone therapy and its relationship to your cardiovascular system, breast cancer, your reproductive organs, and other health conditions. We also provide a bunch of information on non-hormonal treatments (both conventional treatments, such as medications, and non-conventional routes like herbal therapy and acupuncture) for many of the symptoms and conditions facing menopausal women.

Chapter 10

The Basics of Hormone Therapy

Hormone therapy (HT) may not be right for everyone, but it definitely can relieve many menopausal symptoms and prevent or postpone diseases that afflict women later in life.

Some women swear by HT, some women fear it, and some women are currently experimenting with hormone therapy to figure out the types, combinations, and dosages that are right for them to maximize the protective effects of HT and minimize the risks. (Arguments about the potential risks of HT abound, and we discuss them thoroughly in many chapters of this book, particularly Chapter 15.)

But many women aren't comfortable enough with their level of knowledge about HT to make up their minds about where they stand on the subject. If you're a member of this group, that's okay. Trying to understand the full significance of the choices presented by your medical advisors can be frustrating and confusing. In this chapter, we explain the various hormones and hormone therapy regimens and how they work.

Hormones are powerful, and you should understand what you put in your body.

Defining Hormone Therapy

Some experts don't like to include the term *replacement* when referring to hormone therapy because *replacement* implies that a *deficiency* exists. Producing lower levels of hormones isn't a disease; it's one of many natural, normal transitions a woman's body makes throughout her lifetime. The simpler and more accurate term for the hormones prescribed during perimenopause and menopause is *hormone therapy*. This term reflects a more progressive attitude about menopause.

Hormone therapy is a program of estrogen and progestin (both of which are classifications of hormones that support reproductive functions and other internal systems), which are administered to relieve perimenopausal and menopausal symptoms and lower the risk of osteoporosis, colorectal cancer, and perhaps Alzheimer's disease. Doctors often prescribe hormones during *perimenopause* (the years before menopause when women experience many of the symptoms — hot flashes, sleeplessness, and so on — associated with menopause). After menopause, you can gradually discontinue use of hormone therapy.

Physicians who recommend hormone therapy after menopause do so because it protects against osteoporosis and relieves *urogenital atrophy* (thinning and drying of your vagina or ureter) exacerbated by low levels of estrogen. In many women, the hormone boost also improves mood and the sense of well-being. Some women remain on hormone therapy for upwards of 20 years; others discontinue use after only a few years. You and your doctor can work together to determine whether hormone therapy is right for you and how long you should remain on it.

Women without a uterus (women who have had a hysterectomy) may take estrogen replacement therapy (ERT — so as not to confuse it with the extraterrestrial character). When estrogen is used alone, it's called *unopposed estrogen therapy* because progestin isn't included to oppose the effects of the estrogen.

From the 1950s through the 1970s, doctors routinely prescribed *estrogen* (the female hormone responsible for giving you breasts, a curvy figure, a menstrual period, and more) by itself to treat menopausal symptoms. As the incidence of endometrial cancer in menopausal women climbed, researchers noticed that menopausal women were more prone to endometrial cancer if they were taking estrogen therapy. Researchers also found that if you take *progesterone* (the hormone that causes you to have a period and slough off the endometrial lining during your reproductive years) for a few days, the risk of endometrial cancer drops.

Here's why the addition of *progestin* (the synthetic form of progesterone) reduces the risk of endometrial cancer: Estrogen stimulates growth of the *endometrium* (uterine lining) to make a nice soft nest for a fertilized egg. Women were designed to shed the endometrial lining if the egg isn't fertilized. That way you clean out the nest each cycle to get ready for the next ovulation. Shedding the endometrium also serves another purpose because an occasional precancerous cell may be located among the endometrial lining. Stimulated growth month after month causes the occasional precancerous cell to multiply along with the normal cells. If you don't shed these precancerous cells, you're liable to develop endometrial cancer.

So researchers tried giving women progestin (the female hormone that causes changes in the uterus) for a few days. Just like in a natural cycle, when the progestin levels rise and then fall, the endometrial lining sheds — getting rid of any precancerous cells.

Menopausal women who don't take hormone therapy and women who are still menstruating (and shed their endometrial lining each month) rarely have problems with endometrial cancer.

Taking estrogen without balancing (or opposing) it with progestin is referred to as *unopposed estrogen therapy*. Women who've had a hysterectomy are really the only women who should receive estrogen alone. Without a uterus (which is removed during a hysterectomy), their chances of developing uterine cancer drop to zero. (Take a look at the "Unopposed estrogen therapy" section later in this chapter for more info.) For most other women, a combination of estrogen and progesterone is necessary.

Slaying the symptoms

For some women, perimenopausal symptoms are so severe that they truly interfere with their family lives, careers, self-esteem, or happiness.

Physicians have routinely prescribed hormone therapy to alleviate symptoms of perimenopause, such as hot flashes, vaginal dryness, disrupted sleep, mood swings, and so on, and it works fabulously. (Check the Cheat Sheet or Chapter 3 for a full rundown of perimenopausal and menopausal symptoms.) Despite studies that suggest that there are health risks associated with hormone therapy, many women wouldn't want to go without hormone therapy because perimenopausal symptoms threaten their enjoyment of life.

People around the world have developed alternative therapies to alleviate the symptoms associated with perimenopause, and women in the Western world have started to choose alternatives to traditional hormone therapy. (Check out Chapter 16 for a rundown of alternative approaches.)

Preventing serious health problems with hormone therapy

Thanks to improvements in nutrition and healthcare, women living in the United States and Canada today may live into their eighties and nineties. Consider this: In 1900, North American women could expect to live to a ripe old age of 50 (barely into menopause). But today the average lifespan is nearly 80 years (way beyond menopause). If you're an average woman (or better than average), you definitely want to consider shifting to a healthier lifestyle. And you may want to consider hormone therapy.

Here's why: Estrogen keeps the engine that is your body running smoothly, and you're going to be driving this car for quite some time (unlike the women in historical times who only drove the car while it was new). Think about how you maintain your car. It's one thing to be a quart low on oil when you're driving a couple miles to the grocery store — it may not do much damage. But taking a 2,000-mile trip when you're down a quart of oil is a completely different story. Your engine will burn up long before you reach the end of your journey. Just like you routinely check your oil level and add to it when necessary (before noticing a problem, we hope), you may need to intervene with medicine even when you're not sick to keep your body running smoothly.

The health problems standing in the way of staying active and comfortable are related to the fact that women produce lower levels of estrogen after becoming menopausal — which can be 20 or more years of your life. Low levels of estrogen can lead to health issues such as

- ✔ Osteoporosis
- ✔ Hardening of the arteries
- ✔ Heart disease (including heart attack and angina)
- ✔ Increased risk of some cancers
- ✔ Memory changes

Preventing some of these debilitating diseases and conditions is one of the reasons women elect to take hormone therapy. But most women first start hormone therapy to relieve the annoying symptoms of perimenopause, such as hot flashes, and continue to take it for years.

Given the results of the recent Women's Health Initiative study and reassessments of other studies, hormone therapy seems to be only one leg of a four-legged stool. Hormone therapy provides greater benefit to women who also eat a healthy diet, get regular exercise, and visit their doctor regularly. We examine the benefits and risks of hormone therapy and the ramifications of long-term use in greater detail in Chapter 15.

Ticking through the Therapies

Every woman's body is different, and you can choose from a variety of regimens and many different types of hormones. We know that trying to get a handle on all the available hormones and therapies on the market can be overwhelming. So, in this section, the goal is to help you understand the different types of treatment programs women use and why they use them.

Estrogen plays such a large role in so many of your body's functions that compensating for the decreased production levels that menopause brings is a key component of most hormone therapies.

During menopause and beyond, the perimenopausal symptoms generally begin to subside, and the bigger concern is preventing, delaying, or treating health issues such as bone loss, cancer, and not-so-hot blood cholesterol levels.

Unopposed estrogen therapy

Unopposed estrogen therapy refers to a treatment program in which you receive only estrogen without any form of progesterone.

Doctors only use unopposed estrogen if you have no uterus (you've had a hysterectomy) because taking estrogen without progestin can lead to endometrial cancer.

If you have a history of blood-clotting problems (deep vein thrombosis), be careful about the types and doses of estrogen you use. In general, blood-clotting problems are associated with high dosages of estrogen — particularly with smokers. Today, physicians are trained to prescribe low-dosage estrogen. Whether or not you smoke, your physician generally starts you on the lowest dosage available and moves you to a higher dosage only if the lowest dosage doesn't relieve your problems. Low-dosage estrogen reduces your risk of blood clotting.

Some evidence shows that the estradiol form of estrogen is less likely to contribute to clotting problems than the conjugated types of estrogen. Because patches don't send estrogen to the liver where it stirs up trouble, they seem to be the delivery method of choice to avoid clotting problems.

If you have an existing problem with liver or gallbladder disease, discuss these conditions with your doctor before using any type of estrogen. Patients with uncontrolled blood pressure shouldn't start on high doses of estrogen.

Treatment methods

Your doctor will evaluate your symptoms and hormone levels in order to establish an appropriate dosage. You may take an estrogen pill every day or use a patch that you apply to your abdomen once or twice a week (the exact timing depends on the brand and your doctor's recommendations). Creams you apply to your skin (like you apply a moisturizer) are also available.

Benefits

Taking unopposed estrogen boosts the amount of estrogen circulating in your bloodstream. This boost alleviates a variety of symptoms including

- **Headaches:** Estrogen increases blood flow by relaxing blood vessels.
- **Hot flashes, heart palpitations, and anxiety:** A drop in estrogen triggers your brain to release adrenaline, which makes your heart race and your blood vessels dilate.

✔ **Interrupted sleep:** This state of affairs is often the result of hot flashes. Estrogen alleviates hot flashes and increases serotonin production, so you're able to sleep through the night.

✔ **Memory lapses:** Estrogen promotes communication among nerve cells in the brain.

✔ **Mood swings and irritability:** Estrogen increases serotonin production.

✔ **Vaginal dryness and atrophy, frequent urination, and urinary incontinence:** Estrogen acts as a moisturizer to your urogenital tissues, keeping them pliable enough to avoid these problems.

Estrogen also has beneficial effects on bone maintenance, cholesterol levels, blood pressure, clotting factors, and the health of your blood vessels and heart tissue. (Check out Chapter 2 for more information.)

Taking unopposed estrogen also eliminates the premenstrual-symptom-like side effects of bloating, breast tenderness, and similar symptoms caused by progesterone.

Side effects

If you take estrogen alone without progesterone or progestin, you won't have periods after menopause like you would with combination hormone therapy (see the "Combination therapy" section later in this chapter). Your *endometrium* (lining of your uterus) will continue to thicken and create quite a buildup. The buildup can lead to endometrial cancer (sometimes referred to as uterine cancer).

Other side effects from estrogen include breast fullness or tenderness, an increase in *triglycerides* (a type of fat in your blood), and an increase in blood pressure. These side effects can often be reduced or eliminated by decreasing the dosage or switching from the pill form of estrogen to an *estradiol* (active estrogen) patch that you place on your skin.

Sometimes side effects reflect a reaction to a dye or some inert (inactive) ingredient in an estrogen tablet and can be eliminated by switching from the pill to the patch. These side effects may include joint aches, muscle aches, skin irritation, and a burning sensation that accompanies urination.

Cautions

Anyone who still has a uterus shouldn't use unopposed estrogen therapy because of the risk of endometrial cancer. If you have a history of breast cancer or you're experiencing undiagnosed vaginal bleeding, your physician won't prescribe unopposed estrogen therapy even if you've had a hysterectomy.

For women who have had a hysterectomy and have a family history of breast cancer, the answer isn't so clear. You and your doctor should have a frank discussion to decide if this type of therapy is for you.

You may have assumed this little pearl of wisdom, but we want to mention it anyway: Stay away from estrogen therapy if you're pregnant.

Combination therapy

Combination therapy means taking a combination of hormones as opposed to taking only estrogen. Generally, combination therapy consists of a combination of estrogen and progesterone (or the synthetic form of progesterone called *progestin*). Some women need to boost their *androgen* (male hormone) levels as well, so testosterone or another male hormone may be part of the combination. Some women who experience a low libido take a small dose of testosterone in their "hormone cocktail."

Combining progesterone with estrogen provides the benefits of estrogen while reducing the risk of endometrial cancer that taking unopposed estrogen can heighten. The only bad part is that progestin/progesterone may slightly reduce some of the benefits of estrogen. The sole purpose for including progestin in hormone therapy is to reduce your risk of endometrial cancer. If you have a uterus and you elect hormone therapy, your doctor will put you on some form of combination hormone therapy.

The combination products on the market contain varying doses of both estrogen and progesterone/progestin.

Treatment methods

Combination therapy has a couple basic regimens for you and your medical advisor to choose from. If you're interested in hormone therapy and you don't have a medical history that rules it out, you and your doctor will review some information to decide what's right for you.

Combination hormone therapy comes in two basic forms: Cyclic and continuous combination therapy. And cyclical combination therapy has a few different options you can choose from. Each form has its own set of indications that make it the right choice.

- ✓ **Cyclic combination therapy:** With this form, you're taking estrogen and progestin in a cycle — generally the first part of the cycle involves estrogen; the second involves progestin. This combination will trigger a period because the progestin tells your uterus to shed the endometrial lining.

"But I thought menopause meant that you don't have a period," you say? Well you're right. You're not technically having a menstrual period; you're having vaginal bleeding. Drugs, not ovulation, trigger the periods that come with hormone therapy. Cyclic hormone therapy causes most women to have predictable vaginal bleeding, which can continue for years.

There are two common cyclic combination programs:

- In one regimen, you take estrogen every day of the month and estrogen and progestin together for the last 10 to 14 days of every cycle.

- In the other cyclic combination regimen, you take estrogen everyday for 25 days of the month and progestin for 10 to 12 days. You take no medication for 3 to 6 days each month. You can expect to bleed when you're not taking the medication. Some people refer to this regimen as *sequential combination therapy* because you take the estrogen and progestin in a sequence.

✔ **Continuous combination therapy:** With this form of therapy, you take estrogen and progestin together every day. This approach seems to provide these benefits:

- Lower risk of endometrial cancer

- Cessation of periods after six months or a year

- Fewer progestin-related side effects in some women (see the following "Side effects" section), especially bleeding

Pills and patches on the market today combine the two hormones making them easy to take. But some women who are sensitive to progestin experience fewer side effects when using a progestin cream and taking estrogen as a pill or patch. If you're bothered by side effects, talk with your doctor about experimenting with different dosages or forms to make you more comfortable.

Some women on combination therapy don't like the side effects they feel on the days they take progesterone. Don't stop taking progesterone/progestin without consulting your doctor, and take it for the exact length of time prescribed by your doctor. Taking just estrogen can lead to endometrial cancer. (For more information, see the "Unopposed estrogen therapy" section earlier in this chapter.)

Certain progestins are derived from testosterone and can help women who complain of low libido (sex drive) during and after menopause. The generic name for this progestin is *norethindrone.* Although norethindrone reduces many of the progestin side effects, it's not recommended for women with high LDL-cholesterol or trygliceride levels. Like estrogen, you can take testosterone via creams, regular pills, pills you hold under your tongue, and vaginal suppositories. Doctors most commonly prescribe low-dosage skin creams and pills because these forms cause your body to absorb the testosterone more slowly, helping you avoid side effects caused by rapid shifts in your hormone levels.

Benefits

Combination therapy should give you the best of all worlds — the benefits of estrogen (and perhaps testosterone) without the risks of endometrial cancer.

Continuous hormone therapy causes fewer side effects in women who are several years beyond menopause than in younger women. Plus, continuous hormone therapy causes fewer premenstrual-like symptoms than cyclic hormone therapy. For those of you who are tired of tampons, one-third of women stop bleeding when they start the continuous combination therapy, many women stop monthly bleeding after two to three months, and most women stop monthly bleeding after one year of therapy. But proper dosages and delivery forms are needed to curb the side effects of progestin.

Women who have problems with their libido often find that a bit of testosterone in their hormone therapy gives it a boost.

Side effects

Some women have a hard enough time tolerating human progesterone, and tolerating its synthetic cousin, progestin, is no easier. The progesterone/progestin can cause many premenstrual-syndrome-like symptoms, including

- ✔ Acne
- ✔ Bloating
- ✔ Depression
- ✔ Weight gain

Cautions

Women with a history of breast cancer should not take hormone therapy, and those with a family history of breast cancer should carefully consider the risks. Also, women shouldn't take hormone therapy to prevent coronary artery disease or reduce the risk of heart attack, according to the recent results of the Women's Health Initiative study.

Women who have heart disease, uncontrolled diabetes, high blood pressure, high triglyceride levels, fibromyalgia, or depression aren't good candidates for continuous combination therapy because taking progestin every day often exacerbates these conditions.

Selective Estrogen Receptor Modulators (SERMs)

Meet the stealth bombers of the hormone therapy world. SERMs are manufactured designer drugs that target specific types of estrogen receptors (those areas that welcome and use estrogen) while blocking estrogen receptors in other parts of the body. SERMs don't contain estrogen. They stimulate estrogen receptors in the bone, brain, and cardiovascular system, but block the receptors in the breast and uterus.

This way, the drugs provide the benefits of estrogen to specific parts of the body without the drawbacks — the biggest drawback being the increased risk of breast cancer. The U.S. Food and Drug Administration (FDA) has approved two SERMS for use in the United States:

✔ **Tamoxifen:** Designed for women who have been stricken with specific types of breast cancer to prevent further recurrence, tamoxifen is generally used in conjunction with other forms of treatment (such as surgery or chemotherapy). But researchers also have found that it provides benefits similar to hormone therapy — lowering blood cholesterol and improving bone density.

✔ **Raloxifene:** Approved by the FDA for treatment and prevention of osteoporosis, raloxifene builds bone and slows down the destruction of bone during the bone maintenance process. Raloxifene, like tamoxifen, seems to provide a bit of improvement in blood cholesterol, lowering bad cholesterol and total cholesterol slightly. This SERM doesn't increase your risk of endometrial or breast cancer.

Treatment methods

Both tamoxifen and raloxifene are available in pill form and should be taken as directed by your physician.

Benefits

SERMs may reduce bone loss in menopausal women, but not as well as estrogen. SERMs reduce the risk of breast cancer in women if taken for no more than five years. Unlike combination hormone therapy, SERMs have no negative effects on blood lipids, so they won't raise your triglyceride or LDL-cholesterol levels.

A lot of research is still ongoing, and new types of SERMs are on their way. Targeting specific estrogen receptors for enrichment seems to be a very promising way to help women stay comfortable and healthy during and after menopause.

Side effects

Unfortunately, SERM use brings some side effects:

✔ Insomnia

✔ Slight increased risk of endometrial cancer (with tamoxifen)

✔ Significant hot flashes

SERMs are beneficial to your blood cholesterol, but they do increase the risk of blood clots in your veins and lungs and may lead to strokes.

Cautions

Anyone at risk of cardiovascular problems should avoid SERMs. Also, women with hot flashes don't tolerate SERMs well because they tend to make the symptoms worse

Pills, Patches, and Pomades: A Smorgasbord of Delivery Options

Over the years, scientists have worked hard to provide hormone therapy that maximizes the benefits and minimizes the side effects and inconveniences. The result of all this effort is a smorgasbord of choices. Basically, you have three paths to choose from to deliver hormone therapy to your bloodstream: your mouth (pill), skin (patch or cream), or vagina (cream, gel, or ring). A fourth hormone-delivery path, muscle (injection), exists but isn't used for hormone therapy.

The various delivery systems offer choices to suit the personal and physiological preferences of a diverse group of women. You and your doctor can experiment to find the delivery methods and dosages that are most effective for you.

In the following sections, we list the types of delivery systems available and the benefits and drawbacks of each. We also go through the different types of hormones used in hormone therapy one by one and indicate how they can be delivered.

Popping pills

Taking pills by mouth is a very traditional way of ingesting medication, so understanding and correctly performing the procedure is very easy. Getting the exact dose that the doctor ordered is also simple because the prescribed dosage is already loaded in the pill; plus the frequency is written on the label. Hard to get this one wrong.

But, when you reach the 60 or 70 mark, you may be taking additional medications. For example, by that time in their lives, many women are taking a multivitamin, extra calcium, high-blood-pressure medication, maybe something to strengthen their bones, and on and on. An additional pill in the parade can be a pain.

Pasting on a patch

Patches deliver drugs through the skin. In the old days (two or three years ago), bulky patches with a sometimes-skin-irritating reservoir of alcohol delivered the hormone. Today's patches are known as *matrix patches* because the hormone is actually incorporated in the adhesive that attaches to the skin. The patches currently on the market are much smaller, thinner, and less likely to irritate your skin than the patches of days gone by.

Patches have some advantages:

✔ You put them on once or twice a week.

✔ They deliver a constant supply of hormone so you have more consistent hormone levels in your blood.

✔ They're easier on your liver and digestive tract than pills are because they bypass these areas of your body and go straight into your bloodstream.

Really, the only problem you may have with a patch is that it could irritate your skin. Not many women have a problem with that though.

Applying creams

Vaginal lining responds very quickly to treatments applied directly to the area. Some women like vaginal creams because they deliver the hormones localized in a small area.

If you're treating vaginal dryness or atrophy yet worry about breast or endometrial cancer, a cream may be a good choice. For example, an estrogen cream relieves vaginal dryness and atrophy but doesn't increase your risk of breast cancer because the dosage is low and the estrogen stays put.

Creams are effective at treating your vagina, but they do nothing for your hot flashes, mood swings, bones, or blood cholesterol.

Cream applicators can be cumbersome to load and can make the whole process difficult and inexact. You may get more or less of a dose than you expected, and inevitably, you lose some cream from the vagina after the application. So you're never really sure exactly how much cream you've truly applied and how much you've lost. You may feel like putting a bit more in the applicator to compensate, but you don't know how much extra to add. Because applying creams is cumbersome, some women just quit doing it or don't apply the cream on a proper schedule.

New vaginal estrogen tablets have recently come on the market. These tablets are easy to apply, give a precise dose, and make less of a mess. One of these tablets is about the size of a baby aspirin, and you insert high into the vagina with an applicator like you'd use for a tampon, only narrower. The pill dissolves slowly inside your body and releases small amounts of estrogen. You administer these pills about twice a week.

Slipping on a ring

This ring doesn't go on your finger; you place it in your vagina. Rings are fairly new in the United States, but women in Europe have been using them for quite a while.

The doctor usually inserts the flexible, hormone-containing ring initially; after that you can change it — usually every 90 days. The ring slowly delivers an even supply of hormones to your bloodstream. The dosage is very low, so it doesn't stimulate growth of the endometrial lining.

Don't worry: The ring is out of the way. But some women do have a problem tolerating the ring because they have short or narrow vaginas. Also, you can pop it out if you're straining on the potty. But, if you're okay with a diaphragm, the ring isn't that much different.

A ring is a great option for women with vaginal and urinary tract symptoms, but it doesn't provide all the other health benefits of estrogen such as relief of perimenopausal symptoms and improved bone maintenance.

Rejecting injections

Although hormones are available as shots, they're not used in hormone therapy. Physicians generally prescribe hormone shots just prior to surgery for patients who are about to have their ovaries taken out. Injections keep the hormone levels in the patient's bloodstream from crashing after the surgery.

Searching for Sources

For those of you who like to exchange recipes, here's a quick overview about how drug companies make these hormones. In the following sections, you can see that hose folks in white lab coats have been very resourceful in finding ways to create hormones.

Synthetic versus natural hormones

Are you the type of person who only eats natural, organic foods? Do you opt for fresh veggies over the canned variety? Do you grab bottled water because of those funny floaties or that weird smell in your water at home? If you answered yes to any of these questions, you may be wondering how to maintain this level of purity in your hormones too.

Well, how can we put this? Deciding what's *natural* when it comes to hormone therapy can be difficult. Like beauty, natural (hormone therapy) is in the eye of the beholder. You can look at *natural* a couple of ways:

- ✔ Natural can mean similar to what you already have in your body. In the laboratory, scientists can replicate the exact molecular structure of human hormones. The results are identical to human hormones but without the stray bits that exist in all animal hormones. So these hormones have the same structure as natural human hormones, but they're made in a lab, so they're synthetic.

- ✔ Natural can also mean coming from nature (you know, plants and animals). Some hormones are derived from plants but need to be modified to produce a beneficial effect in our bodies. Other hormones come from animals. So, these natural hormones come from nature, but they're not *natural* to humans.

So, *natural* isn't really a good term for describing the hormones used for hormone therapy. In the next section, we give you the source of the hormone — you get to decide whether you consider it natural or not.

Estrogen

Some really clever scientists have found a variety of sources from which to make estrogen. Over the years, trying to get the right type and amount of estrogen into your body has been quite a challenge for the guys and gals in lab coats.

Before we get started with the recipes for hormone therapy, a quick reminder about the in's and out's of estrogen may be in order. Three types of estrogen exist: estrone, estradiol, and estriol. We mention this fact because all types of estrogen are not created equal. Here's a brief estrogen primer (the whole story is in Chapter 2):

- ✔ **Estradiol** is the biologically active type of estrogen and the most potent form of human estrogen. It's a player in hundreds of bodily functions.

- ✔ **Estrone** isn't the workhorse that estradiol is; estrone is more like the warehouse variety of estrogen that's stored in your body fat. It can be turned into estradiol, but only in premenopausal ovaries.

✔ As for **estriol,** fuggetaboutit — in this context anyway. Estriol is mostly found in pregnant women.

All right. Now that that's taken care of, here are the sources of estrogen that scientists have come up with:

✔ **Conjugated equine estrogen:** Made from the urine of pregnant horses. Some of the most-prescribed estrogens used in hormone therapy are conjugated equine estrogens. This type of estrogen has the least amount of estradiol, but it delivers lots of estrone and a significant amount of *equilin,* an estrogen used by horses. Although equilins are great for female horses, doctors occupy both sides of the fence on the subject of whether equilin is beneficial to human females. Conjugated equine estrogen is available in pill, injection, and cream form.

✔ **Estradiol estrogen:** Derived from soybeans and/or wild yams. These estrogens are chemically identical to human estradiol estrogen. Estradiol estrogen is available in every delivery method — pill, cream, ring, and patch. (Check out the "Pills, Patches, and Pomades: A Smorgasbord of Delivery Options" section earlier in this chapter for more info.) In fact, it's the only type of estrogen used in the patch.

✔ **Esterified estrogen:** Made from soybeans and/or wild yams (sometimes referred to as Mexican yams). Esterified estrogen provides high levels of estrone and much lower levels of estradiol estrogen, but it has been shown to help maintain bone and improve perimenopausal symptoms and lipid profiles in the blood. Esterified estrogen is available as a pill.

✔ **Estropipate:** Also known as *piperazine estrogen sulfate.* Available as a pill or cream, this synthetic form of estrogen is chemically similar, but not identical, to human estrone.

A drawback of estropipate: It may actually aggravate pain in women who have muscle- or bladder-pain syndromes.

✔ **Micronized estradiol:** Provides women with the same type of active estrogen (estradiol) that the ovaries produce naturally. The estradiol is produced synthetically (in the lab) from soybeans.

Micronization means that the particles are small enough to be absorbed into your bloodstream before your digestive system destroys them. So here we go with the "What's natural and what's not?" discussion. Micronized estradiol is made from a "natural" plant, but technicians tweak it in the lab so that your body can use it. You take this estradiol as a pill.

Some doctors claim that using a form of estrogen that's molecularly similar to human estradiol is no more beneficial to women than estrogen products derived from pregnant mares; others claim that it makes all the difference in the world.

Progestin

Most of the side effects attributed to hormone therapy are the result of the progestin, but progestin protects you from developing endometrial cancer. Because every woman's body is different, you may need to do some experimenting to figure out which progestin is right for you.

Adding progestin to the hormone therapy mix does seem to reduce the benefits estrogen can have on your cholesterol levels and increase changes to your mood.

There are three types of progestin on the market:

- **Progesterone:** Identical to the human hormone produced by the ovary in premenopausal women. Progesterone is available as a pill and as a vaginal gel.

- **Medroxyprogesterone acetate (MPA):** Originally used to regulate menstrual cycles. Doctors now prescribe it in hormone therapy to slough off, or thin, the endometrial lining at the end of a course of estrogen, thereby reducing the risk of endometrial cancer.

- **Progestin derived from testosterone:** Includes norethindrone and norethindrone acetate progestin. They seem to have fewer side effects than MPA and offer a boost to the libido in some women. These progestin aren't recommended for women with high cholesterol or low HDL (the "good" cholesterol) levels. Norethindrone and norethindrone acetate are available either as pills or patches.

Combinations of estrogen and progestin

For convenience sake, you may want to combine estrogen and progestin into a single pill or patch.

A couple brands on the market contain conjugated estrogen with a progestin called medroxyprogesterone acetate (MPA). The U.S. Food and Drug Administration approved MPA for women having trouble with their periods. MPA helps prevent the *endometrium* (uterine lining) from thickening too much and helps regulate periods. MPA is useful in combination hormone therapy because it inhibits the over-thickening of your endometrium, so it lowers your risk of endometrial cancer.

Conjugated estrogen and MPA is a commonly prescribed combination therapy and can be administered as either sequential courses of estrogen followed by progestin or as continuous combination therapy (see the "Combination therapy" section earlier in this chapter).

Today, new combination therapies use a progestin derived from testosterone, *norethindrone acetate,* instead of MPA because it causes less vaginal bleeding. You can get a combination therapy in both patch and pill forms. The combination patch administers the estradiol form of estrogen and norethindrone acetate. Many women like the patch because you don't have to remember to take a pill and it's convenient to have both hormones delivered in a single patch.

Androgens

When we talk about *androgens* (male hormones), we're mainly talking about testosterone.

You may need to include androgens (most likely testosterone) in your hormone therapy for a couple of reasons. If you've become menopausal due to surgery (removal of your ovaries), your androgens may take a nosedive very quickly. You may want to bump your androgens up because they help bone maintenance and libido. Women who experience natural menopause may need androgens in the regimen because estrogen supplements may decrease the amount of physiologically active testosterone in your bloodstream (which could lower your libido and lessen muscle tone).

Using too high a dose of testosterone has some side effects: acne, oily skin, hair loss, unwanted hair, and a deeper voice. Rest assured that prescribed dosages are rarely high enough to trigger these side effects.

Doing the Dosing

The guideline that every doctor uses is this: Use the smallest dose possible to alleviate symptoms and health risks while minimizing the side effects. That said, women react to hormone supplements very differently. No one knows why a particular regimen causes one woman to experience side effects and another to sing its praises from the rooftop.

Your doc will review your personal medical history, your family medical history, and the results of your physical examination and lab work. He'll also want to consider what conditions or problems you're trying to overcome or prevent. (For example: Are we talking about lessening perimenopausal symptoms or preventing osteoporosis after menopause?) Share your personal preferences and prejudices with your doctor at this time as well. (Do you have a hard time swallowing pills? Do you forget to take medicine? Are you determined to throw away the tampons as soon as possible? These kinds of issues.)

During perimenopause, some women experience symptoms that make life absolutely miserable. Doctors may try prescribing a hormone therapy regimen in these cases. Here are the standard schedules for hormone therapy:

- ✔ **Cyclic:** Take estrogen daily and add progestin for 10 to 14 days per month.

- ✔ **Cyclic/Sequential:** Take estrogen for 25 days each month and progestin for 10 to 12 days each month. No medication is used for 3 to 6 days per month. Vaginal bleeding is expected during the period when no medication is taken.

- ✔ **Continuous:** Take estrogen and progestin daily. You generally have no vaginal bleeding after a few months of using continuous hormone therapy (which is why many women like this regimen).

- ✔ **Patch:** Apply a *transdermal* (skin) patch twice a week (or as directed) to an area of the body not exposed directly to the sun.

If you have issues with your libido, your doctor takes it into the equation when prescribing hormone therapy. Convenience is also an issue. Convenience considerations include how many other medications you take (do you really want to take more pills or use a patch), the cost, and how anxious you are to quit bleeding every month. As far as the last issue goes, *sequential/cyclical therapy* (taking estrogen for part of the month and progestin another part of the month) results in continuing your periods for some time, but *continuous combination therapy* (taking both estrogen and progestin at the same time every day) generally stops your periods. SERMs also eliminate your periods.

In Table 10-1, we outline the hormone dosages generally recommended for many of the common hormone therapies available in the market. The numbers refer to dosage for the days you take the associated drug. Your doctor may need to do some experimenting with these different products to find the right one for you — one that will eliminate your symptoms while producing the few side effects. (Remember that *mg* stands for *milligrams* as you check out the table.)

Most doctors start out using standard doses but then customize dosages to the individual. With hormone therapy, one size doesn't fit all. So your doctor may take a number of blood samples to figure out where your hormones are and try to administer dosages that will get your hormones to an appropriate target level (see the "Targeting your hormone levels after menopause" sidebar in this chapter).

Table 10-1   Suggested Starting Doses for Hormone Therapies

Generic Chemical Name	Product Name(s)	Common Dose
Oral Estrogens		
Conjugated equine estrogen	Premarin	0.625 mg
Esterified estrogen	Estratab	0.625 mg
Estropipate	Ogen; Ortho-Est	1.25 mg
Oral Combination Estrogen/Progestin		
Conjugated equine estrogen/MPA	Prempro	0.625/2.5 mg daily
Estrogen Skin Patches		
Estradiol	Alora; Climara	0.05 mg
Estradiol	FemPatch	0.25 mg
Estradiol	Vivelle	0.0375 mg
Combination Estrogen/Progestin Skin Patch		
Estradiol/norethindrone acetate	CombiPatch	0.05/0.14 mg daily
Estrogen Creams		
Conjugated equine estrogen	Premarin vaginal cream	1.0 gram — 0.625 mg
Estradiol	Estrace vaginal cream	1.0 gram — 0.1 mg
Estrogen Rings		
Estradiol	Estring vaginal ring	1 ring
Progestins		
Medroxyprogesterone acetate (MPA)	Cycrin; Provera	2.5 mg
Oral micronized progesterone	Prometrium	100.0 mg
Megestrol acetate	Megace	20.0 mg
Norethindrone	Micronor; Nor-QD	0.35 mg
Nortethindrone acetate	Norlutate	5.0 mg

Targeting your hormone levels after menopause

So just how much active estrogen do you need pulsing through your body to keep you healthy and comfortable for the years to come?

Most people in the field agree that estrogen levels after menopause don't need to be as high as they are in premenopausal women. Women can obtain good energy, mood, sleep, and memory levels when blood levels of estradiol are above 90 to 100 pg/ml. (That's picograms per milliliter. A picogram is one-trillionth of a gram.) This is quite a bit lower than the premenopausal estradiol level of 200 pg/ml typical in the first half of your period and the 300-to-500-pg/ml level during ovulation.

Estradiol levels below 90 pg/ml result in the typical hot flashes, interrupted sleep, mood swings, and other annoying menopause symptoms. Below 80 or 90 pg/ml, you risk bone loss and cardiovascular issues. So your target is to get your estradiol levels up to 90 or 100 pg/ml. What constitutes a normal testosterone level is not as easily agreed upon. Normal levels are between 15 and 75 ng/dl (nanograms per deciliter). Some experts feel the target level is 40 ng/dl to maintain a healthy sexual appetite and energy level.

Chapter 11

Hormone Therapy and Your Heart

· ·

· ·

*U*ntil the results of the Women's Health Initiative (WHI) study were released early in 2002, most medical folks thought that the one certainty in hormone therapy (HT) was the benefits it brought to your heart. Although there's still no question that estrogen lowers your risk of heart disease and keeps your blood cholesterol healthy *during your reproductive years,* HT may not be the godsend for menopausal women that most experts thought it was.

The research into whether hormone therapy actually makes for a healthier cardiovascular system has been all over the place. Researchers have been studying this issue for decades, but some of the studies are small or biased in their selection of people to study. So doctors and medical groups were all drawing their own conclusions as to which study to believe, resulting in medical opinions on the topic that have been all over the board.

You need to seriously consider cardiovascular issues because, whether you're talking about stroke, high blood pressure, or heart attack, more women die of cardiovascular disease than men.

This chapter helps you understand the what's and how's behind the beneficial effects hormone therapy has on your cardiovascular system and fills you in on the drawbacks. We also apply the findings of the WHI study to each area we examine. With this info in hand, you can make better long-term decisions about how to live a healthy life during perimenopause and menopause and how to cope with cardiovascular risks that increase with age. (But, before you make any decisions, check out the other HT chapters in this book too — Chapter 10 and Chapters 12 through 17.)

Meeting the Players: Hormones and Your Heart

As far as your sex hormones go, estrogen, progestin, and testosterone play different roles in your cardiovascular system, so you probably want to know what they do for a living. You're in luck! In the following sections, we outline what these hormones do for your blood, blood vessels, and heart before menopause. The trick to hormone therapy is to find the right levels of hormones that provide protection to the heart without raising the risks of heart attack, stroke, or blood clots (or breast cancer).

The star: Estrogen

Because estrogen protects the cardiovascular system, women have about a ten-year grace period for developing heart disease when compared to men. In fact, most of the cardiovascular benefits attributed to hormone therapy are due to the protective nature of estrogen.

Take a look at how estrogen works on your cardiovascular system:

- Decreases triglycerides, which you don't want to be high
- Increases HDL levels
- Reduces fibrinogen, which can cause blood clots
- Reduces the risk of blood clots
- Relaxes artery walls to help dilate blood vessels and avoid spasms
- Improves blood flow in the coronary arteries
- Reduces the buildup of plaque in your coronary arteries
- Decreases blood pressure when taken via a skin patch

But it's only fair to list the negative effects estrogen replacement can have. You can avoid these problems by paying attention to the type of estrogen you take and the delivery mechanism you use to administer it.

- Can cause clots (deep-vein thrombosis) at high levels
- Increases triglycerides when taken as a pill
- A skin patch doesn't effect HDL and LDL levels for six months

Yes, different methods of delivery can produce different results. (For more details on the advantages and disadvantages of different estrogen-delivery forms, check out Chapter 10.)

Continuously reviewing your hormone-therapy regimen throughout your life is very important. Your health conditions can change, which may lead you to make a change in your program.

The supporting actor: Progesterone

Progesterone's main function is to prepare your body for pregnancy. When progesterone levels peak, most women feel bloated and ravenously hungry. Your breasts often feel tender and enlarged. If your egg isn't fertilized, progesterone levels drop, you have your period, and these symptoms go away.

So why in the world would anyone knowingly make women take this hormone after they finally rid their systems of it? Researchers and doctors haven't always understood the benefits of progesterone on normal body functioning. (With all the uncomfortable symptoms progesterone causes, is it any wonder that the white coats looked past the positives?) But recently, medical people discovered that estrogen, when taken alone, can increase a woman's risk of endometrial (uterine) cancer. So, doctors have added *progestin* — synthetic progesterone — to nearly all HT programs to lower the risk of endometrial cancer of the uterus. The discovery that progestin can limit the cancer risk associated with estrogen-only therapy is a huge benefit for menopausal women. (Women who have their uterus surgically removed don't receive progestin because they no longer have to worry about uterine cancer.)

Although progestin reduces the risk of endometrial cancer, it has some negative effects on your cardiovascular system. In particular, progestin

- ✓ Lowers HDL ("good" cholesterol) levels.
- ✓ Increases triglycerides (very-low-density lipid — nearly all fat).
- ✓ Lowers your sensitivity to insulin, which affects your ability to process glucose. This effect is of great concern to diabetics.
- ✓ Tends to make women's bodies store fats instead of breaking them down.

With the variety of progestins on the market today, some of these problems have gone by the wayside. Doctors can vigilantly scrutinize your regimen to make sure that you get the proper dosage, the proper delivery form, and the proper type of progestin. For more information on the advantages and disadvantages of various hormone regimens, take a look at Chapter 10.

Your doctor must perform an individual assessment of you and your needs to determine the right answers to your HT-regimen questions.

The assistant: Testosterone

Women's bodies naturally produce testosterone, a so-called male hormone. When given with *estradiol* (the active form of estrogen), testosterone helps relax and dilate the blood vessels, improving the flow of blood. If testosterone is given on its own with no estradiol, it seems to have the opposite effect, promoting plaque buildup on vessel walls.

Testosterone is touchy stuff, so work with your doctor to make sure that your hormone therapy is promoting a healthy balance in your hormone levels. When women take testosterone along with estrogen, some of these negative effects of testosterone seem to be reversed according to newer studies. If testosterone is part of your HT regimen, your doctor will religiously monitor your blood cholesterol and modify treatment as needed.

Understanding the Significance of the Women's Health Initiative Study

The *Women's Health Initiative* (WHI) study, the one that stirred the HT debate early in 2002, is much better designed than previous studies. It used about 16,000 participants and employed solid research methods. There's only one problem: The WHI only studied one type of hormone therapy — conjugated equine estrogen combined with MPA (medroxyprogesterone acetate) progestin. Although physicians commonly prescribe this type of hormone therapy, experts disagree about whether it's the safest or most effective form of hormone therapy.

The results of the WHI study are important, and they scientifically document the effects of this particular course of therapy on women's health. We think that these new results are important enough that we provide you with their conclusions throughout this chapter. But we also provide you with information on the use of unopposed estrogen and research from other studies evaluating the use of estrogen and progesterone. For those of you who were worried that the WHI study would answer all the questions concerning hormone therapy, we just have to turn to our old friend Mike Myers and say, "Not!"

Skimming the Fat: Hormone Therapy and Your Blood

Heart disease (often called *coronary heart disease*) is often caused by hardening of the arteries or coronary artery disease. Over the years, fat can get deposited on the walls of your blood vessels and attract other substances that eventually get capped by a calcium layer. This process, called *atheriosclerosis,* causes your arteries to thicken and impedes the flow of blood through your veins. This state of affairs can raise your blood pressure, forcing your heart to pump harder.

A chunk of the *plaque* (the goop formed by fat and other substances) can break off and clog an artery, causing a heart attack or stroke. A stroke can also be caused by blood clots forming unexpectedly because of the presence of a greater-than-necessary amount of clotting chemicals in your blood. These clots can get stuck in a blood vessel that feeds your brain (stroke), in a deep vessel the feeds your heart (deep vein thrombosis) or lung (pulmonary embolism), or in your heart itself (heart attack). All in all, the blood, blood vessels, and heart comprise your *cardiovascular system,* and a problem in one area can lead to trouble in another.

To avoid blood problems, keep your total cholesterol, LDL ("bad" cholesterol), and triglyceride levels low and keep your HDL ("good" cholesterol) levels high. This advice is important for anyone who's concerned about staying heart healthy. But, when the topic at hand is predicting cardiovascular risks for women, forget what you've heard about total cholesterol as the main event. The focus is on your triglycerides — keep them low — and your HDL levels — keep them high. (Chapter 5 tells you everything you need to know about cholesterol.) Here's what the medical community knows about the effects of hormone therapy on your blood.

Women's Health Initiative findings

The results published to date don't indicate whether conjugated estrogen and MPA progestin had any negative or positive effects on blood cholesterol.

Unopposed estrogen

A variety of studies indicate that estrogen (used as a pill or patch) without progesterone can provide a variety of benefits. Estrogen

  ✔ **Decreases LDL levels:** Estrogen helps get rid of some of the "bad" cho-lesterol in your blood by increasing the amount of LDL your liver breaks down, so that more LDL gets purged from your arteries. Estrogen pills are more effective than patches at this job, but both work over time.

  ✔ **Increases HDL levels:** HDL cholesterol is the type of cholesterol that can carry excess fat out of your bloodstream and back to your liver for reprocessing.

> ✓ **Improves the metabolism of carbohydrates:** Your body gets some help digesting sugars, which helps lower your risk of diabetes.
>
> ✓ **Helps maintain healthy blood clotting:** Like Goldilocks, you want it just right. Blood clots protect you from bleeding, but if you clot too easily, you can have a stroke or develop artery-clogging deposits (atherosclerosis).

By helping maintain healthy triglyceride and cholesterol levels in your blood, estrogen lowers your risk of developing atherosclerosis, which is a major cause of angina, stroke, heart attacks, and other problems.

You can only use unopposed estrogen if your uterus has been removed.

Estrogen plus progestin

Do you see all the wonderful benefits estrogen brings about? Well, add progestin and the scenery changes. When added to estrogen in hormone therapy, progestin tends to muffle the benefits of estrogen. But hormone therapy does slightly improve blood cholesterol, raising HDL levels slightly and lowering LDL levels slightly. Women using hormone therapy generally have better blood cholesterol levels than women who don't use anything.

Healthy blood helps make a healthy you.

Keeping the Pipes Clean: HT and Your Blood Vessels

Your heart stays alive and receives nourishment via your *coronary arteries,* blood vessels that branch from the aorta and deliver oxygen to your heart muscles. If your coronary arteries get messed up, you *will* have trouble.

Hormones play a major role in maintaining healthy blood vessels, including your coronary arteries. Your hormone levels must be balanced to keep your blood vessels open and the blood flowing smoothly through them. The following sections make the heart and hormone connection.

Avoiding clogs

When your blood contains more fat (LDL cholesterol) than your HDLs can comfortably haul away, some of the fat may be deposited inside your blood vessels. Trouble begins when your coronary arteries get clogged with fat and a gunk known as *fibrinogen* (a substance which helps blood clot). After a while, the accumulation forms a crust called *plaque* (fat plus other substances form the foundation, and calcium caps the top of the pile). As plaque builds, it narrows the blood vessels and constricts the flow of blood to your heart — atherosclerosis is the diagnosis at this point.

The studies have this to say about benefits and harms of hormone therapy on atherosclerosis.

Women's Health Initiative findings

The results published to date don't provide analysis of negative or positive effects of conjugated estrogen and MPA progestin on atherosclerosis.

Unopposed estrogen

Estrogen not only helps your body maintain a healthy and balanced cholesterol profile (see the "Skimming the Fat: Hormone Therapy and Your Blood" section earlier in this chapter), it also shines up your blood vessels by

- **Protecting the coronary arteries from plaque buildup:** It prevents the walls of the arteries from thickening and keeps plaque deposits from forming in the arteries.

- **Keeping the vessels dilated:** It performs this trick by relaxing the vessel walls.

- **Decreasing plaque formation:** This is accomplished by preventing the adherence and formation of inflammatory cells to the vessel walls.

Estrogen plus progestin

The jury is still out on whether adding progestin to the equation diminishes estrogen's positive effects on blood vessels. None of the studies that took a look at this question are very good.

The Nurses' Health Study does indicate that progestin didn't alter estrogen's beneficial effects, but a study on monkeys showed that progestin added to estrogen blocked blood vessel dilation. (We're rooting for the nurses.)

Controlling the pressure

Hypertension, also known as high blood pressure, has *no symptoms* — that's why it's called the silent killer. As its nickname implies, hypertension is serious stuff. *Blood pressure* refers to the force created in your blood vessels as you heart pumps blood through your body. When your blood pressure rises, your heart has to pump harder to move blood through the tensed-up vessels, putting the vessels under even more pressure. The increased pressure can damage the walls of your arteries and start the process of *arteriosclerosis* (fat and other gunk build up on the walls of your arteries). (For more information on high blood pressure, see Chapter 5.)

High blood pressure is a killer because it forces your heart to work harder, and it can contribute to *coronary artery disease* — disease in which your blood vessels become hard and scarred with plaque and lose their flexibility.

Women's Health Initiative findings

The Women's Health Initiative researchers haven't released any information on positive or negative effects for hypertension in women using conjugated estrogen and MPA progestin hormone therapy.

Unopposed estrogen

The benefits outlined in this section are based on a number of studies that have been conducted using estrogen therapy alone (on women with no uterus). Estrogen can positively impact your blood pressure and the health of your blood vessels by

- **Dilating arteries and other blood vessels in your body:** When arteries become bigger, blood flows more efficiently.

- **Improving blood flow in your coronary arteries:** This benefit is associated with taking estrogen via a pill that dissolves under your tongue.

- **Enhancing the release of nitric oxide:** The release of nitric oxide relaxes the blood vessels. We all know that everything just seems to flow more smoothly when we're relaxed, and that general principle goes for your blood vessels too. Is anything worse than tense and irritable blood vessels?

Estrogen plus progestin

Sorry to say, but the medical community just doesn't have much research to turn to when looking for the effects that taking estrogen and progestin has on hypertension.

Keeping a clear head

People suffer from several different types of stroke, but the one that we're concerned about due to its relationship to menopause and hormone therapy is ischemic stroke. *Ischemic stroke* is caused by an obstruction in an artery, which restricts the flow of blood — and the oxygen it carries — to the brain. The obstruction can be a piece of plaque that broke off from the wall of your artery or a thickened artery wall caused by arteriosclerosis.

A stroke literally suffocates the part of the brain nourished by that clogged artery, impairing the functions that part of the brain directs. Deprived of oxygen, that section of the brain can die, which leads to some type of permanent debilitation. Strokes occur suddenly and, generally, without warning. The first indication may be the loss of some motor function.

Estrogen is thought to lower your risk of stroke because it provides so much protection to your blood and blood vessels (see preceding sections in this chapter). By keeping the pipes clean and flexible, blood is able to flow without obstruction to your brain, thereby lowering your risk of ischemic stroke. Here's what the latest research tells us about hormone therapy and stroke.

Women's Health Initiative findings

The use of conjugated estrogen and MPA progestin actually increased the risk of stroke for women in this study. This risk is probably attributable to the study's determination that during the first year of using this particular type of hormone therapy, the risk of *deep vein-thrombosis* (DVT — blood clots in veins that empty into the heart) and *pulmonary embolism* (blood clots in the lungs) triples when compared to women who aren't using any form of HT.

But you have to realize that under normal circumstances, deep-vein thrombosis effects only 4 out of 10,000 women. Tripling this figure means that 12 women out of 10,000 would develop DVT. It's all a matter of perspective (unless, of course, it happens to you). The increased risk of these dangerous blood clots may be the reason the risk of stroke goes up with use of this type of hormone therapy.

Unopposed estrogen

Estrogen is thought to lower your risk of stroke because of the protective effects it has on your blood vessels and your blood's ability to clot properly. Check out the "Controlling the pressure" and "Skimming the Fat: Hormone Therapy and Your Blood" sections earlier in this chapter for the positive effects of HT on your blood vessels and your blood's ability to clot, respectively. But studies are mixed in their findings, and some results show increased risk of DVT and stroke even among women who use only estrogen.

Estrogen plus progestin

Another large study, the Nurses' Healthy Study, also found that hormone therapy (estrogen and progesterone) increased the risk of stroke in the first two years of use. After two years, the risk seemed to drop back down to a risk level corresponding to the risk women not using hormone therapy face.

Oiling the Pump: HT and Your Heart

The changes that menopause brings have a large impact on your heart, so it makes sense that hormone therapy has a large effect also.

Slowing the pace

A fluttering heart doesn't always signal new love. Many women experience heart *palpitations* (a pounding, racing heart) for the first time during the change.

Palpitations can indicate a variety of cardiovascular problems and should be taken seriously. Check these symptoms out with your primary care physician.

When your estrogen levels drop, as they do during the change, your brain sends out adrenaline in an attempt to spur on estrogen production. Your heart responds to this adrenaline surge by pounding.

The effects of hormone therapy on heart palpitations aren't really on the radar screen of scientists investigating the benefits and harms of hormone therapy. We do know that hormone therapy reduces perimenopausal symptoms, and heart palpitations are considered symptoms (as long as they're not indicative of more serious cardiovascular problems).

Keeping angina away

Angina can feel like you have a weight on your chest. We know, you're already carrying the weight of the world on your shoulders. Is it any wonder that it slips to your chest during menopause? Everything else seems to be drooping! Although some women feel angina even when they do nothing, most women feel the pressure only when they exercise.

You feel pressure because your heart isn't getting enough blood. When you exercise, spasms cause your coronary arteries to tighten, which restricts the flow of blood to your heart. In response, your heart screams to get your attention, and you feel chest pain.

Estrogen has a soothing effect on blood vessels and reduces spasms. Yet, again, angina isn't really in the center of the hormone-therapy-research spotlight. Doctors don't prescribe HT just to help you get rid of angina.

Avoiding the big one

The medical name for a heart attack is *myocardial infarction* (sometimes abbreviated as MI). A heart attack is caused by a blockage in one or more of your coronary arteries. This blockage can be a blood clot or a plaque deposit that breaks from a vessel, flows through the bloodstream, and ends up clogging an artery. Blockages can restrict blood flow to your heart and cause either a heart attack or the death of heart tissue (heart disease).

Women's Health Initiative findings

The WHI study found that heart attacks actually increased 29 percent for women using conjugated estrogen and MPA progestin. But, although the risk of having a heart attack increased, the incidence of dying from one didn't. Based on this information, some doctors are removing patients from hormone therapy. Others are taking more of a wait-and-watch attitude, especially given that these results are out of whack with a number of other studies.

Unopposed estrogen

Estrogen improves blood flow in your coronary arteries by dilating the blood vessels, helping your body continue to eliminate plaque inside the vessels, and maintaining healthy clotting.

Estrogen plus progestin

If you pull together information from all the other scientific studies (excluding the WHI) that look at coronary heart disease, heart attack, and hormone therapy, results show that coronary heart disease is lower among women using hormone therapy. However, when researchers looked deeper into the situation, they found that exercise and alcohol use were the real factors that made the difference, not the hormone therapy, so the results are far from definitive. Look for a lot more research on the effects of hormone therapy and your heart to take place in the near future.

Chapter 12

Hormone Therapy and Breast Cancer

In This Chapter

▶ Recognizing your breast-cancer risks

▶ Debating the benefits of HT and the risk of breast cancer

▶ Choosing an HT regimen with breast cancer in mind

*I*s hormone therapy (HT) risky business in terms of breast cancer? Medical types have suspected that a link between estrogen and breast cancer exists and have researched the suspected link for over 60 years. Reports place estrogen at the scene of the crime time and again, but no conclusive evidence absolutely demonstrates that estrogen is the guilty party. And, if estrogen is one of the perpetrators, some research results claim that it may not act alone. In this chapter, you can find out what researchers know for sure and what they're pretty sure they don't know about HT and the risk of breast cancer.

Beginning with Breast Basics

Breast tissue and fat are the two main components of the breast. You no doubt already know about fat, so that subject needs no further explanation. But breast tissue may be a relative stranger.

Breast tissue is composed of sections called *lobes*. Lobes are made up of *lobules*, which produce milk when you breast feed. *Ducts* carry milk from the lobules to the nipple. Why are we explaining all of this? Because cancers tend to form either in the lobules or in the ducts. Figure 12-1 illustrates the parts of a breast.

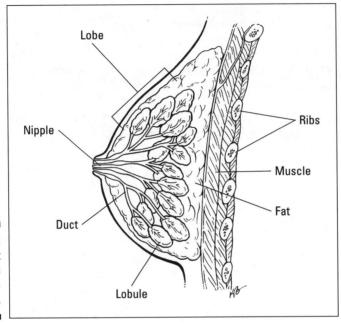

Figure 12-1:
The breast
and its
compo-
nents.

Defining Breast Cancer

Whether breast cancer forms in the lobules or the ducts, it begins when cells divide and grow at an abnormally fast rate. The cells morph into odd shapes and start clumping together to form cancerous (*malignant*) tumors.

What triggers this process? Researchers know that it takes a *mutation* (a freak act of nature that affects the basic building blocks of cells) to get things going, but no one knows how the initial cells become mutated. Most researchers feel that a *carcinogen* (a cancer-causing agent) in the environment serves as the trigger. There are two main types of breast cancer and one condition that can lead to cancer:

✔ **Carcinoma *in situ*:** Technically, this is pre-cancer. *In situ* (which means *in place*) refers to the fact that the cancer cells haven't spread beyond a very restricted area (usually a breast duct or lobule). Carcinoma *in situ* is like a breast-cancer early-warning sign. Basically, your doctor will keep an eye on things because you may get breast cancer in the future.

✔ **Invasive ductile cancer:** This type of cancer starts in the ducts and spreads to surrounding tissues.

✔ **Invasive lobular cancer:** This type of cancer starts in the lobes and spreads to surrounding tissues.

Both invasive ductile and invasive lobular cancers can move through the breast tissue into your blood vessels, thereby gaining access to your entire body. When this happens, the cancer is said to have *metastasized,* or spread.

Treating cancer is much easier when it's confined to your breast. That's why early detection is so very critical.

Taking Care of Your Breasts

You probably already know about the importance of performing a monthly breast self-exam and getting a regular mammogram. The following sections tell you why these two simple tests are so vital to your breast health.

Examining your breasts every month

The American Cancer Society (Internet: www.cancer.org) recommends that you examine your breasts for lumps and bumps every month after you reach the age of 20. And your doctor should do a breast exam as part of your yearly gynecological visit.

The American Cancer Society makes performing self-exams very easy by printing self-exam guide cards you can hang in your shower. The cards show you how to perform a breast exam and what you should look and feel for. Ask your gynecologist for a card or give the American Cancer Society a call (phone: 800-ACS-2345) and ask a representative to send you one.

The most common symptom of breast cancer noticeable during a self-exam is a hard, immovable lump in your breast, which may or may not be painful. Sometimes the skin that stretches over the lump looks thick or indented; sometimes it looks dimpled like an orange peel. You may also notice that your nipple leaks a dark fluid or turns inward. If you notice any of these signs, contact your doctor.

Sometimes a lump you feel in your breast isn't cancerous. Breast lumps can occur as the result of several breast conditions. (For more information on breast conditions, take a look at *Women's Health For Dummies,* by Pamela Maraldo and the People's Medical Society, published by Wiley Publishing, Inc.).

Making time for mammograms

Although you may see articles every year or so questioning the necessity of mammograms, most medical folks say, "Just do it." Mammograms are relatively painless, cost effective, and fast.

Have your first mammogram around age 35 so your doctor has something with which to compare future mammograms. If you're between 40 and 49, you should have a mammogram every year or two. If you're over 50, do it every year.

We don't want to get political here, but the main reason annual mammograms have come under scrutiny recently is due simply to the cost of screening. Here's a fact: The best chance of surviving breast cancer comes from early detection. Individuals who downplay the importance of annual screenings question whether mammogram screenings actually decrease the *death rate*. The more useful measure of the effectiveness of mammograms is whether regular mammograms increase the *detection rate* of new breast cancers — and they do! If you're a woman in your forties, having mammograms on a regular basis can reduce your chance of dying from breast cancer by about 17 percent. For women between the ages of 50 and 69, regular mammograms can reduce deaths by about 30 percent.

Given a choice, most women would like to prevent long and arduous cancer treatments, which is the other important goal here. Early detection can reduce the numbers of women who have to undergo drawn-out and painful treatments for breast cancer. Mammograms can detect cancers before the cancers reach the size of a lump that you can feel. So, with today's mammogram technology, healthcare providers can identify cancer at an early stage, catching the cancer before it invades the bloodstream and gains access to other parts of your body. Early detection allows doctors to treat breast cancer with a relatively noninvasive and short course of treatment.

Recently, the U.S. government decreed that Medicare would only pay for every-other-year mammograms for women over 55 years of age. Nevertheless, get a mammogram every year. Many churches, community centers, schools, and even grocery stores sponsor mobile mammogram centers that offer mammograms at discounted prices.

Determining Estrogen's Role

Although a great deal of controversy surrounds the why's and how's, nearly everyone agrees that estrogen plays some role in the development of breast cancer. Even the natural estrogen in your body during your reproductive

years increases your risk of breast cancer because it stimulates cell reproduction in your breasts. When it comes to estrogen and menopause, here are
the things most experts agree on:

- ✔ Estrogen is a key promoter of breast-cancer development. So controlling
  estrogen levels in breast tissue should lower your risk of breast cancer.

- ✔ The earlier you begin perimenopause and the shorter your reproductive
  cycle is, the lower your risk of breast cancer because these factors
  decrease you total lifetime exposure to high levels of estrogen.

- ✔ Being overweight (gaining 45 pounds or more after your 18th birthday or
  being 20 percent over your target weight) after the onset of menopause
  increases estrogen levels in your body and can increase the risk of breast
  cancer. (Check out Chapter 18 for more info on determining your ideal
  weight.)

  This risk doesn't apply to premenopausal women who are overweight
  (though extra weight does put you at risk for other health problems).

Assessing Your Risks

The two biggest risks for breast cancer are being female and being over 40.
Both risks are realistically unavoidable, and they both present you with a
whole bunch of positives. So who would want to avoid them?

Breast-cancer risk continues to rise after menopause whether you take
hormones or not. But a number of other factors can also increase your risk
of breast cancer. Some are controllable; some aren't.

Protecting your young

The most effective way to reduce the risk of
breast cancer is to start preventing it at a young
age. We know what you may be thinking: "A lot
of good that does me." But this information can
do you good if you pass it along to a young
woman you care about and it does her some
good.

The period of a girl's life before her childbearing years, even before puberty, is a very critical
time in her development. During this time,
breast tissue is more susceptible to toxins that
can cause cancer later in life. The negative
effects of environmental toxins, radiation, a
high-fat diet, tobacco and alcohol use, and
other risk factors all have a greater impact on a
woman during these crucial years than they do
during other phases of her life.

Recognizing risks you can't control

As frustrating as it is, some breast-cancer risk factors are out of your control. Even your own estrogen appears to heighten your breast-cancer risks (see the "Determining Estrogen's Role" section earlier in this chapter). This section lists the risks you can't do anything about, but you can control other factors (which we cover in the "Recognizing risks you can control" section later in this chapter).

✔ **Age:** Of course it's not fair, but the older you get, the greater your risk of breast cancer. That's an important fact to keep in mind. When you're younger than 40, your risk is quite low. But, after 40, your breast cancer risk increases until you're about 80. The good news is that when you hit 80, your risk of breast cancer actually decreases a bit, as shown in Figure 12-2.

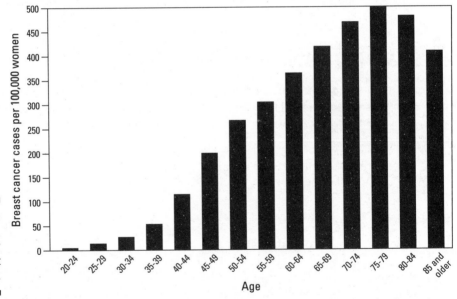

Figure 12-2:
Age as a risk factor for breast cancer.

✔ **Breast density:** Breasts with more breast tissue than fat tissue are comparatively denser. Unfortunately, detecting small tumors in dense breast tissue is more difficult than detecting them in fatty tissue. Gynecologists don't generally examine density, but one major health study found a correlation between breast density and the risk of breast cancer (the denser your breast tissue, the greater your risk of cancer).

✔ **Ethnicity:** In North America, Caucasian women have the highest risk of breast cancer. Ashkenazi Jews are at greater risk of breast cancer than women from other cultures too. No one knows exactly why these Jewish women are at higher risk, but some evidence shows that they have a higher rate of the genetic mutation known as BRCA1 (which we discuss next). Going down the scale, Hawaiian and African-American women have the next highest risk of breast cancer. Latinos, Asian Americans, and Native Americans have the lowest rates of breast cancer in the United States.

✔ **Genetics:** If someone in your immediate family has breast cancer, your risk of breast cancer almost doubles. If both mom and sis have breast cancer, your risk is about 2½ times greater than the risk of a woman without breast cancer in her family.

If you're worried about your family history of breast cancer, you may want to take genetic tests that look for two genetic mutations — BRCA1 and BRCA2 — that leave you more susceptible to breast cancer. However, only about 5 to 10 percent of breast cancers come from inherited genetic mutations.

The letters BRCA stand for *breast cancer.* BRCA1 is a genetic mutation found in people with a family history of ovarian and breast cancer. BRCA2 is a genetic mutation found in people with a family history of male and female breast cancer. Only about 50 to 60 percent of women with these genes actually get breast cancer, and remember that these genes only account for 5 to 10 percent of all breast cancer cases.

The genetic tests are easy, but dealing with the results may be more complicated. Before getting tested, consider what you will do with the information after you have it. Will it simply cause you greater anxiety? Also, find out what measures are in place to guarantee confidentiality so the results are available to you alone and not to insurance companies or other parties.

✔ **Location of fat on your body:** This may sound strange, and you can't really do anything about it, but studies show that if you wear your fat high in your body (around your midsection), your risk of breast cancer is about six times as high as a woman who wears her fat around her hips, thighs, and buttocks.

✔ **Menstrual history:** The later you begin your menstrual cycle and the earlier you begin menopause, the lower your risk of breast cancer. Presumably, your risk of breast cancer is tied to the amount of estrogen you generate during your lifetime.

✔ **"Precancerous" breast tumors:** Receiving a diagnosis of abnormal cell growth, carcinoma *in situ,* for example, increases your risk of breast cancer. (Check out the "Defining Breast Cancer" section earlier in this chapter for more on carcinoma *in situ.*)

Fibrocystic condition of the breast, a condition in which you develop little lumps in your breast tissue (usually seven to ten days before your period), does *not* increase your risk of breast cancer. (For more information on fibrocystic condition of the breast, read *Women's Health For Dummies,* Wiley Publishing, Inc.).

What if you've already had breast cancer?

If you've had breast cancer in one breast, you're at greater risk of developing cancer in the other breast. And victims of ovarian or uterine cancer are at slightly greater risk of breast cancer.

If you've been treated for breast cancer, you already may have decided that hormone therapy is out of the question for you. In fact, the literature that comes with estrogen medications tells doctors not to use them to treat patients with previous or existing breast cancers. But more and more breast cancer survivors are enjoying longer lives; lives that could include osteoporosis, cardiovascular disease, colon cancer, and Alzheimer's disease — all of which hormone therapy may help mitigate. So the choice becomes more difficult.

If menopausal symptoms disrupt your life, talk to your gynecologist. SERMs may be an appropriate therapy for you. (For more information on SERMs, see Chapter 10.)

Recognizing risks you can control

Don't feel forlorn — you can control a lot of the risks associated with breast cancer. To improve your odds by taking control of these factors, you have to evaluate your current lifestyle for behaviors that carry high breast-cancer risks. Check out the following list — maybe you're already living a "breast healthy" lifestyle. In that case, you can give yourself a pat on the back.

- **Alcohol consumption:** Having more than three drinks a week raises your risk of breast cancer. This fact holds true whether you're taking hormone therapy (HT) or not, but it's especially true if you take the conjugated equine form of estrogen. Alcohol raises the level of estrogen (more specifically, the estrone type of estrogen) in your body.

  (For more info about conjugated equine estrogen, check out the "Choosing your HT regimen with breast cancer in mind" section later in this chapter. And for more on all forms of estrogens used in HT, take a look at Chapter 10.)

- **Antioxidants:** Vitamins A, C, E, beta-carotene, selenium, and glutathione are antioxidants that protect the body from premature aging and cancer (see Chapter 18 for more on antioxidants). When taken by menopausal women, these antioxidants lower the risk of breast cancer. Recommended dosages are 400 to 800 IU (international units — a common unit of measure for vitamins and drugs) per day.

- **Dietary fat:** This one is a bit controversial because some studies indicate that high-fat diets increase your risk, other studies are inconclusive, and others show that fat has no bearing on the risk of breast cancer. The studies that show a high-fat diet increases your risk suggest that you have to reduce your total fat intake to 20 percent of the calories you eat each day before you lower your risk.

The type of fat you eat can also affect your risk of cancer. *Saturated fats* (the types of fat you find in animal products such as red meat and cheese) raise your risk of breast cancer. Animal fats also introduce a number of byproducts into your diet that come from the animals' ecosystems, such as pesticides and antibiotics, which are concentrated in the animal fat.

✔ **Exercise:** Studies at the Cooper Clinic tracked patients for more than ten years and found that cancer deaths decreased as women raised their activity levels.

✔ **Pregnancy:** Women who have at least one pregnancy have a lower risk of breast cancer during their *lifetime* than women who have never been pregnant. But you have to read the fine print that accompanies this risk factor because you actually have a slightly higher risk of breast cancer during the ten years immediately following the birth. After ten years or so, your risk of breast cancer drops so that women with one child have a lower risk of breast cancer than women who have never borne a child. In general, the more babies you have, the lower your lifetime risk of breast cancer.

✔ **Weight gain/obesity:** Gaining more than 45 pounds at any point increases your risk of breast cancer. Breast cancer is linked to higher levels of estrogen (especially the *estrone* type of estrogen found in fat). Also, obese women (women who weigh 20 percent more than their target weight) are also at greater risk because they have about 40 percent more estrogen than non-obese women. (Check out Chapter 18 for additional information on weight-related issues.)

Knowing for sure: Tests for breast cancer

If you find a lump in your breast, there are several ways to examine it to see if the lump is something to be concerned about. The type of test your doctor uses depends on the size of the lump and its location.

✔ **Fine needle aspiration:** This procedure can be done right in the doctor's office. The doctor sticks a tiny needle into the lump, drains some fluid, and sends the fluid off to the lab to check for cancerous cells.

✔ **Needle core biopsy:** The doctor performs this test in the hospital as an outpatient procedure. Because the doctor uses a bigger needle, she also uses a local anesthetic to numb the area. The doctor sticks the needle into the suspected problem area, removes some breast tissue, and sends it to the lab to check for cancerous cells.

✔ **Open biopsy:** This surgical procedure is performed in the hospital using anesthesia. The doctor makes a small incision and removes part of the lump or the entire lump, which he then sends to the lab for analysis.

Evaluating the Facts about HT Risks

Everywhere you turn, you may see conflicting stories about the risks of breast cancer when taking hormone therapy (HT). Individuals and groups within the medical community often provide varying opinions depending upon whom you talk to. The source of conflict among the experts is the reliability of the results of studies used to test the breast-cancer/HT connection. Some of these studies used small groups when large groups would have been more reliable. Some of the studies based on large groups of subjects relied on observations or the patients' memories instead of more reliable objective tests. And the type of hormone treatments tested varied from study to study. So, unraveling the connections is often difficult and fraught with disagreement.

If, as Paul Simon sings, there are 50 ways to leave a lover, there are thousands of ways to disagree with research results. In the following sections, we attempt to present both sides of the debate concerning hormone therapy and breast-cancer risk.

The "avoid hormone therapy to avoid breast cancer" argument

The research results that experts who warn of the dangers associated with estrogen and breast cancer rely on include:

- Women who have had both their uterus and ovaries surgically removed before age 40 (and, therefore, stopped producing estrogen before 40 years of age) had a lower incidence of breast cancer. Because your body's own estrogen contributes to the risk of breast cancer, hormone therapy will too.

- The biggest and best controlled study to date, the Women's Health Initiative (WHI) study, clearly shows that women taking conjugated estrogen with MPA progestin are at increased risk of breast cancer after using it for over five years. Also, it seems that the longer you take HT, the greater your risk. (For more information on different types of estrogen and progestin, check out Chapter 10.)

The doctors occupying this camp also argue that most of the conditions that HT regimens are supposed to help can be helped using less risky, non-HT drugs (check out Chapter 17 for more on these medications). The risks associated with cholesterol-lowering and blood-pressure-controlling drugs are less than the risks associated with HT for women who are at risk of heart disease. And non-hormonal drugs that protect bone density are also available.

The "benefits outweigh the risks" argument

Experts who believe that HT benefits outweigh the risks of breast cancer have this to say:

✔ Some well respected doctors, who wanted to set the record straight, recently pulled together all the hormone studies and found that 14 of 18 studies reported no increase in the risk of breast cancer in women who used estrogen at one time or another.

✔ If you look at breast-cancer rates for women not taking HT, the rate of breast cancer is highest among women who have experienced menopause. The conclusion you might draw from this fact is that the incidence of breast cancer rises as you get older, even if you don't use HT.

✔ The 1989 study that got everyone's attention by claiming that HT raised the risk of breast cancer was later corrected to show no meaningful difference in the incidence of breast cancer between the HT and non-HT groups.

✔ A Harvard study that found much higher rates of breast cancer in women who were taking estrogen didn't point out that the increase was only in the group of women who used a certain type of estrogen (conjugated equine estrogen) and also drank alcohol. The group of women who took estrogen but didn't drink alcohol showed about the same incidence of breast cancer as women who didn't take estrogen.

✔ If you compare women on HT with those not on HT, the death rates from breast cancer are very similar. One might expect a higher death rate in women who use HT if it caused breast cancer.

✔ A higher percentage of low-grade, less aggressive breast cancer cases exist among women who take HT versus those who don't. If HT promotes breast cancer, it promotes a less aggressive form.

Interpreting the evidence

The previous sections tell the story of HT and the risk of breast cancer as the medical establishment understands it today. Research continues, and maybe, a less confusing conclusion will be drawn in years to come.

At the end of the day, the HT choice is yours. But here are some things to think about when reviewing all the evidence:

✔ **What are your individual health risks?** If you or your family members have osteoporosis, or dementia, you may be thinking seriously about HT. If you or an immediate family member have had breast cancer, you should be very cautious about the risks of HT and breast cancer. Breast cancer is a terrible disease, but sometimes, people underestimate the consequences of osteoporosis, which HT has been shown to lessen, and dementia, which HT seems to impede. Get the facts on both before making up your mind.

✔ **What can you live with?** When you consider the quality of your life, consider what type of concessions you're willing to make. Combating osteoporosis requires a healthy diet and a regular exercise program, often in combination with medication. Would you be able to stay on track if you had to take medication and increase your exercise to fight osteoporosis? Everyone agrees that estrogen relieves perimenopausal symptoms like hot flashes and all the rest (see Chapter 3). Can you live with these symptoms? Cancer scares all of us, no matter how small the risk, and if we can do anything to reduce the risk of cancer, most of us will do it. But considering the evidence about the links between HT and the risk of breast cancer, how do you evaluate your risk of breast cancer?

✔ **What do you fear most?** Some people dread getting Alzheimer's disease; some fear having a heart attack; and others worry about cancer. Most of us have opinions of what the worst possible illness would be. Use these opinions when considering your alternatives.

Reading your alphabet soup: Results from the WHI on HT and BC

The Women's Health Initiative (WHI), the results of which were published in 2002, is one of the new and improved studies that included tens of thousands of women (a huge study by anyone's standards). The WHI researchers also used some very sophisticated techniques to make sure that the study wasn't biased in terms of the type of women selected to participate. (Participants of all ages, ethnicities, medical histories, and so forth took part.) The results provide terrific hard facts about the use of *the most commonly prescribed HT regimen.*

But here's the problem: You can't necessarily generalize and say that these results are the hard and fast facts about *all the different HT products* used by women. We know that different types of estrogen and progesterone produce different effects. Conjugated estrogens have different effects than estradiol estrogen, and pills work differently than patches (for the details on the differences, turn to Chapter 10). So, if you're using (or contemplating using) conjugated equine estrogen and MPA progestin, be aware that the WHI results show increased risk of breast cancer with long-term (more than five years) use.

Given that research results don't provide an obvious choice concerning HT, you need to look at your own health goals and interpretations of the research results.

Finding the Right HT Program

Over the years, the medical establishment has reached a consensus on the need for different hormone therapy (HT) regimens because women have different hormone profiles, menopausal symptoms, and medical conditions. And certain types of estrogen result in a higher risk of breast cancer than others. In the case of HT, one size fits no one.

Discussing HT and breast cancer with your doctor

Because no clear-cut answers exist about whether HT raises your risk of breast cancer, most doctors try to advise you about the benefits and potential risks concerning HT instead of simply writing a prescription and sending you on your way. If your doctor doesn't present you with a balanced comparison of the benefits and risks associated with HT, ask him to discuss them with you. The HT decision isn't one to be taken lightly, and your doctor should spend time with you to make you feel comfortable about your choices.

Choosing your HT regimen with breast cancer in mind

The type of estrogen that seems to have the greatest correlation with an increased risk of breast cancer is a form known as *conjugated equine estrogen,* which is made from the urine of pregnant horses. (For more information on the different forms of estrogen used in HT, flip over to Chapter 10.) This type of estrogen gives you much higher levels of *estrone* (the inactive form of estrogen) and long-lasting estrogens that seem to bond stronger and longer to the estrogen receptors in the breast.

But to be fair, conjugated equine estrogen is the most widely used and the most widely studied form of estrogen, which may be why it appears to be more closely related to breast cancer than other forms.

Another large study found that the *combination* of estrogen and progesterone increased the risk of breast cancer in menopausal women who had
taken hormones for five to ten years. Critics of the findings suggest that
because the women took the conjugated equine form of estrogen, the risks
were higher for the group. In other words, the results had as much to do
with the type of estrogen the women were taking than the combination of
progesterone with the estrogen.

Take a close look at yourself when you answer the question, "Is HT right for
me?" The role of HT in breast cancer is still unanswered. Despite lots of
research, all we can say is, "We don't know." You need to review all the
available information on breast cancer and HT and then consider your
own medical issues and family history.

Choosing alternatives

If you smoke or use alcohol daily, if you're obese, or if you have breast cancer
in your immediate family, you should definitely discuss HT with your doctor
and discuss possible alternatives to hormone therapy. Think about your medical risks, your values, and your preferences in making your decision.

Chapter 13

Hormone Therapy, Cancer, and Your Reproductive Organs

*H*ormone therapy (HT) has been linked to all kinds of cancers "down there." In some cases, HT is thought to lower the risk of cancer. In other cases, it may increase the risk of cancer. And, in others, it's thought to have absolutely no effect.

In this chapter, we look at cervical, colon (or more accurately colorectal), endometrial (uterine), and ovarian cancers. In each case, we introduce you to the particular cancer and its symptoms, review the screening procedures and tests, discuss the role (or lack thereof) HT plays in connection with each cancer, and perform a quick risk-benefit analysis.

What about breast cancer? Well, because of all the issues that surround that topic, we devote an entire chapter — Chapter 12 — to that type of cancer.

Colorectal Cancer

The colon and the rectum are the last stops on the digestive tract before waste moves out of the body. The first six feet or so of the large intestines is called the *colon;* the last six inches is called the *rectum.* If you're wondering how your body holds six feet of tubing, take a look at Figure 13-1, which shows the location of the colon and rectum.

Though commonly known as colon cancer, the proper name for this type of cancer is *colorectal cancer* because it can occur in either the colon or the rectum.

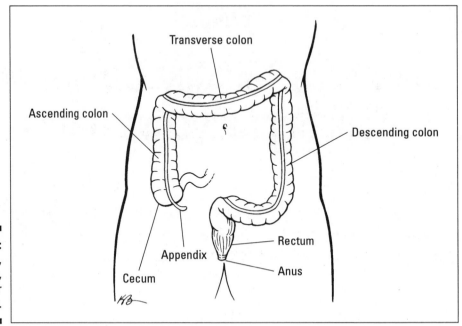

Figure 13-1:
The colon,
rectum,
and other
connections.

Colorectal cancer is a slow-growing cancer that begins as a *polyp* (a small growth) on the mucous lining (*mucosa*) of the colon, as shown in Figure 13-2. Polyps can show up in the colon and be perfectly harmless (asking why is like asking cats why they pounce; they just do). But some polyps have the potential to become cancerous.

One of the most common cancers, colorectal cancer is the third leading cause of cancer death in American women (behind lung and breast cancer). Over 90 percent of cases are found in people over 50 years of age. Colorectal cancer is easily detectable, and you can easily prevent it by making a few healthy lifestyle choices and having regular checkups.

Recognizing the signs

Rectal bleeding and bloody stools are the most common symptoms of colorectal cancer. Additional symptoms include diarrhea, constipation, skinny stools, frequent gas pains, and feeling like you can't completely pass the stool. Some people with this disease lose weight, feel fatigued, or become *anemic* (a condition in which you don't have enough red blood cells to carry oxygen around your body).

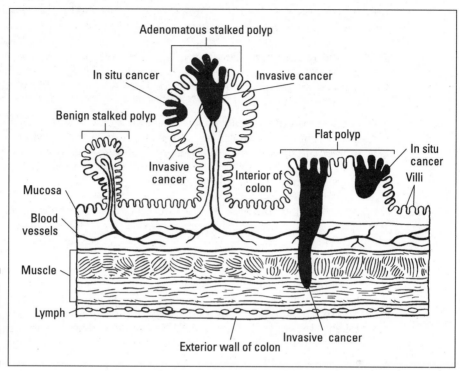

Figure 13-2:
Polyps in the colon may become cancerous.

Finding out for sure: Screenings and tests

A number of screening procedures reduce your risk of colon cancer. Having an annual screening, in fact, is *the number-one way* to reduce your risk of colorectal cancer if you're a woman over age 50. When your doctor checks you out for colorectal cancer, she can look for cancer *and* polyps on the lining of your colon that may become cancerous. Removing any polyps removes some of your cancer risk as well.

Here's why catching polyps early is so important: When colorectal cancer is found before it spreads to other areas of the body, the survival rate is 90 percent. When colorectal cancer spreads, long-term survival rates drop to 9 percent. So getting annual screenings after you turn 50 is well worth the effort.

Generally doctors start out with minimally invasive screening procedures, such as the digital exam and fecal occult test, and move to more invasive procedures only when initial results warrant additional tests. The following tests are generally your first line of defense:

- **Digital rectal exam:** This test is the part of your annual gynecological checkup that you probably look forward to the least. Your doctor inserts a gloved finger into your rectum to check for lumps, bumps, or other changes in the rectum.

- **Fecal occult blood test:** This test is a bit messy, but it really must be done. Some of the newer tests look like some home pregnancy tests — a piece of paper turns a different color if the sample has blood in it. Your doctor takes a sample during your exam and places it on a test card. You know the results immediately.

If blood is found in your stool or the doctor feels something suspicious during the digital exam, the doctor may perform one of these procedures to further check things out:

- **Colonoscopy:** You normally get a mild sedative for this test. During a colonoscopy, your doctor inserts a scope into your colon, which allows her to carefully examine the walls of your colon and rectum (yes, all six feet or so). With the neat technology doctors have today, they may even take pictures of your colon walls and polyps (if any are found). Usually your doctor removes any polyps that she finds and has them examined by a lab for evidence of cancer.

- **Sigmoidoscopy:** Doctors normally sedate patients before performing this test. Your doctor inserts a thin scope about 10 to 12 inches into your rectum through which he can see any polyps or damaged areas in your colon and take a sample if necessary.

- **Barium enema:** You may hear folks refer to this test as a *lower GI series*. It's not used very often; colonoscopies and sigmoidoscopies are more common. This procedure involves a barium enema and a technician taking a series of x-rays of your colon and rectum. The barium highlights your colon — particularly any polyps or growths. If you have growths, your doctor will probably perform a colonoscopy or sigmoidoscopy, depending upon where the growths are located.

Determining the role of hormone therapy

For reasons unknown (though most researchers suspect estrogen plays the role of the heroine here), hormone therapy lowers your risk of colon cancer. In fact, you reduce your risk of colon cancer by more than one-third while you take hormone therapy.

The risk reduction only exists while you stay on hormone therapy; the protection diminishes after you stop taking it.

Assessing your risks

Some of the factors that raise your risk of colorectal cancer are

- **Age:** Why does this one always show up as a risk factor for just about everything? It's here again because over 90 percent of colorectal cancer patients are over the age of 50. With each decade after 50, your risk doubles.

- **Diet:** We're talking about diets high in animal fats here. Eating red meat frequently (once a day) can double your risk of colon cancer. Fat is the culprit. Animal fat not only is the saturated, unhealthy variety of fat, but toxins also tend to gather in it. If the animal you're eating was exposed to pesticides or other toxins before it became dinner, you get those poisons when you chow down.

- **Family history:** Genetics play a role in colorectal cancer (and many other cancers as well). If you have one or more family members with colon cancer, your risk doubles.

    A couple other genetic syndromes bump up your chance for colorectal cancer, but they're quite rare. What are these other syndromes? Things like *familial adenomatous polyposis* and *hereditary nonpolyposis colorectal cancer* to be specific. Aren't you glad you asked?

- **Lifestyle:** Is going from the couch to the freezer to grab a bowl of ice cream your idea of a brisk walk? If it is, listen up. You can cut your risk of colorectal cancer in half by getting out and exercising. Whether you bike, jog, or simply walk (no your couch-to-freezer regimen doesn't count), you lower your risk. Turn to Chapter 19 for the skinny on exercise.

Endometrial (Uterine) Cancer

Cancer of the uterus is usually referred to as *endometrial cancer* because the cancer usually starts in the *endometrium* — the lining of the uterus. Take a look at Figure 13-3 to see the uterus and nearby organs.

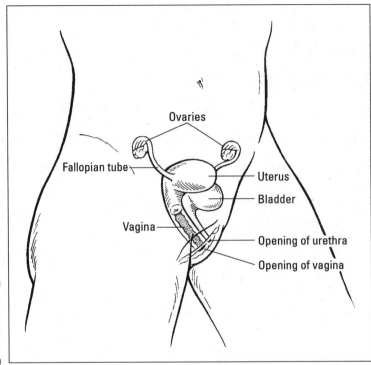

Figure 13-3:
The reproductive organs.

Ovaries

Fallopian tube

Uterus

Bladder

Vagina

Opening of urethra

Opening of vagina

Endometrial cancer is one of the most common reproductive cancers in the North America, but it's readily detected — 75 percent of cases are caught before the cancer moves beyond the uterus — and treatment is very effective.

The endometrium is very responsive to changes in hormone levels. Like many cancers, endometrial cancer occurs when mutant (cancer) cells grow abnormally fast. Too high a level of estrogen or continued high levels of estrogen over a sustained period of time cause cells in the endometrium to continue to multiply. If a mutant cancer cell or two are among those normal endometrial cells, the estrogen will stimulate cell growth and allow the cancer cells to multiply along with the normal cells. The occasional cancer cell is usually not a problem because it gets flushed away during your period, so it doesn't have a chance to proliferate. But, with high levels of estrogen (stimulating cell growth), these cancer cells can multiply.

If you don't have a uterus because you've had a hysterectomy, you don't need to worry about endometrial cancer because you don't have endometrial tissue.

Looking at the life of the endometrium

When you have your period, the surface of the *endometrium* (the lining of the uterus) is sloughed off, leaving just a thin layer of endometrial cells. At the end of your period, your ovaries bump up the level of estrogen production.

In response to the higher levels of estrogen, the endometrium thickens. You then ovulate, at which time your ovaries produce even higher levels of estrogen along with progesterone. The estrogen continues to tell the endometrium to grow thicker, and the progesterone causes it to develop blood vessels and store nutrients for nurturing a fertilized egg.

If there's no fertilized egg, the progesterone and estrogen levels drop, your period begins, and you slough off much of the endometrium. If the egg is fertilized, you continue to produce high levels of progesterone.

Recognizing the signs

Most cases of endometrial cancer are caught and caught early enough to cure because the symptoms are so obvious. Any of these symptoms are a signal to see your doctor:

- ✔ Bleeding after menopause
- ✔ Irregular vaginal bleeding
- ✔ Unusual spotting between periods

Pain and cramping are generally *not* an early symptom of this type of endometrial cancer. (But, after endometrial cancer develops, it can invade the blood vessels and spread to other organs causing this type of pain.) And some women experience no symptoms at all.

Finding out for sure: Tests

A number of tests can identify endometrial cancer:

- ✔ **Dilation and curettage:** Often referred to as a *D&C,* this test entails scraping tissue from the lining of the uterus for examination. Doctors usually perform this procedure under anesthesia in the operating room.

- ✔ **Endometrial aspiration or biopsy:** With this test, the doctor removes a tissue sample from the lining of the uterus for examination. Endometrial aspirations can be done in the doctor's office. Usually there's no need for painkilling medication beyond ibuprofen.

✔ **Hysteroscopy:** This test involves the doctor inserting a special micro-scope into the uterus to examine the lining — usually under anesthesia in the operating room.

✔ **Ultrasound:** Using sound waves, the doctor is able to create images of the uterus lining with this test. Ultrasounds are done in the doctor's office, and they're relatively painless. An ultrasound wand is inserted into the vagina so the technician can get a clear view of the uterus and lining.

Determining the role of hormone therapy

This one is pretty simple. The higher the dose of estrogen and the longer the duration of high estrogen levels, the higher the risk of developing cancer in your uterus.

In the 1970s, after women had been taking estrogen replacement therapy without a *progestogen* (a term that encompasses both synthetic and natural forms of progesterone) for years, medical folks noticed that the incidence of endometrial cancer was three to eight times higher among women taking estrogen compared to women not taking it.

After studying the problem, doctors realized that without a progestogen, the lining of the uterus continued to thicken unchecked. So now, hormone therapy includes a progestogen to routinely flush the lining of the uterus through vaginal bleeding (cyclical hormone therapy) or to keep the lining from growing (continuous hormone therapy). For more info on the different types of hormone therapy, turn to Chapter 10.

If you don't have a uterus because you've had a hysterectomy, you don't need progesterone in your hormone therapy (as women with a uterus do) to balance the estrogen to avoid endometrial cancer.

Assessing your risks

Because an imbalance in hormones (particularly estrogen and progesterone) increases your risk of this type of cancer, things that alter your hormone levels can raise your risk:

✔ **Age:** Over 95 percent of women with endometrial cancer are over 40 years of age. The rate of endometrial cancer rises between the ages of 40 and 70 and then drops around age 80.

✔ **Estrogen:** Taking estrogen replacement therapy without progesterone increases the risk of endometrial cancer. But at least one study showed that women who used a combined therapy of estrogen and progestin had a lower risk of endometrial cancer than women who did not use HT at all.

✔ **Obesity:** Fat tissue produces estrogen. Women who are 20 percent over their ideal weight walk around with sustained, high levels of estrogen because their body fat produces it. Fat is the primary producer of estrogen in women after menopause. (For more on weight-related issues, see Chapters 18 and 19.)

If you're obese, losing weight reduces your risk of endometrial cancer.

Women who have never had a baby have never experienced long periods of high progesterone levels. So obese women with no prior pregnancies are at an even higher risk of endometrial cancer.

Birth control pills actually *lower* your risk of endometrial cancer. Women who use the pill for more than two years reduce their risk by about 50 percent, and women who use the pill for more than five years reduce it by 80 percent.

Cancers Unaffected by Hormone Therapy

We're including information on a couple of other cancers of the female persuasion even though hormone therapy has no known effects on a woman's risk of developing these cancers or her ability to recover from them.

So why are they here? We primarily include them so we don't leave you wondering how hormones affect these reproductive organs. After all, only women have these organs, so questioning the effects of hormone therapy on them is natural.

Also, we think a book that addresses health issues facing menopausal women would be incomplete without at least discussing these cancers.

Cervical cancer

Cervical cancer is the same thing as cancer of the cervix. A *Pap smear* usually detects this form of cancer quite early. Because a virus (human papilloma virus, to be specific) is associated with cervical cancer, practicing safe sex can prevent it.

HT is not known to have any impact on cervical cancer.

Ovarian cancer

The *ovaries* hold your *oocytes* (seeds that develop into eggs over the course of a woman's reproductive years) and produce sex hormones throughout your life. Take a look at Figure 13-3 to locate the ovaries. Ovarian cancer originates from cells in the ovary — both the egg-making cells and the lining of the ovary.

Cancer of the ovaries (known as *ovarian cancer*) kills silently. Few tangible symptoms warn women of this disease until the tumor has spread beyond the ovary. Even in the later stages of the disease, the symptoms are pretty general — bloating, nausea, vomiting, constipation, or frequent urination. A lot of things can cause these problems — a bad piece of fish, too much wine, the flu, you name it. Ovarian cancer is deadly, but fortunately, it's very rare.

Some researchers suggest that ovarian cancer is related to frequency of ovulation during your lifetime. Every time you ovulate, you get a little tear in the ovary wall. The cells of your ovary repair the tear by dividing rapidly. This wear and tear in connection with the rapid cell division needed to repair the damage may be the source of ovarian cancer. Given this explanation, women who have taken birth-control pills (either the old-time high-dose pills or the current low-dose pills) may actually lower their risk of ovarian cancer because the pill suppresses ovulation.

If you've had no pregnancies, you may have a higher risk of ovarian cancer than women who have been pregnant simply because you've never experienced prolonged periods of time during which you haven't ovulated.

Recognizing the signs

Most of the symptoms of ovarian cancer are quite generic — in other words, they can apply to any number of conditions. Many women first notice bloating in their abdomen. Of course, this symptom can be easily confused with some of the symptoms of premenstrual syndrome. Other women experience nausea, vomiting, or gas that just won't go away despite changes in diet. Frequent urination and constipation are also possible symptoms as are abdominal or pelvic pain. The problem is that the symptoms usually aren't present until the disease has entered an advanced stage.

Finding out for sure: Tests

If you experience any of the symptoms listed in the "Recognizing the signs" section, consider getting a pelvic exam and then a blood test that looks for the presence of CA125. *CA125* is an ovarian cancer *antigen,* meaning that it's a substance that causes the body to fight ovarian cancer. If your CA125 levels are high, you may have ovarian cancer. Unfortunately determining the meaning of high CA125 levels is tricky. Sometimes elevated levels show up if you have endometriosis, ovarian cysts, or fibroids or if you're pregnant. Because this test produces a lot of false positives, some doctors don't use it very often. But you should take this test during your annual gynecological screening after you turn 50.

Just because your CA125 levels aren't elevated doesn't necessarily mean you definitely don't have ovarian cancer — 20 to 30 percent of women with ovarian cancer don't have elevated CA125 levels. Likewise, having elevated CA125 levels doesn't mean that you absolutely have ovarian cancer, but it's a reason to further explore the cause of the results.

Given that the symptoms are so disarming and the disease is so deadly, CA125 provides doctors with one point of information in trying to diagnose this disease early. Plus, a CA125 test may identify some more-*benign* (not cancerous) medical conditions such as endometriosis and fibroids. All in all, if you're having symptoms, taking this test is a good idea. Medical folks use a variety of other tests (in addition to a pelvic exam and CA125 test) in their attempts to detect ovarian cancer:

- **CAT scan:** The *CAT* in *CAT scan* stands for *computerized axial tomography.* This procedure lets your doctor get a graphic image of your ovaries to check for tumors.

- **Laparoscopy:** This is a minor surgical procedure in which the doctor makes a tiny incision in your belly button and inserts a scope to get a better view of your ovaries. This exam is done under a general anesthesia in an operating room on an outpatient basis.

- **Pelvic ultrasound:** With this exam, a sonographer inserts a sounding device into your vagina so he or she can view an image (a *sonogram*) of your ovaries. Tumors can be identified with the sonogram.

Determining the role of hormones

Hormone therapy neither raises nor lowers your risk of ovarian cancer.

Birth-control pills may reduce your risks of ovarian cancer, mainly because they suppress ovulation, not because of the estrogen or progesterone levels in your bloodstream. Using birth-control pills for two years reduces your risk by 40 to 50 percent. Using birth-control pills for five years reduces your risk by 60 to 80 percent.

Fertility drugs that increase the number of eggs released during ovulation or increase the number of ovulations you have over a lifetime can increase your risk of ovarian cancer. Again, it doesn't seem to be the blood hormone levels that create the problem so much as the physical wear and tear of ovulation.

Assessing your risks

Ovarian cancer is fairly rare. It only affects 4 percent of women, most of whom are over 50 years of age. But this form of cancer is quite deadly because it usually goes unnoticed until the advanced stages of the disease.

Certain factors increase your risks for ovarian cancer:

- A family history of ovarian cancer (mother, sister, or daughter) or breast cancer (mother or sister)
- The use of fertility drugs that stimulate the ovaries to release multiple follicles during a single ovulation
- Being over the age of 50
- Having never been pregnant

Chapter 14

Hormone Therapy and Other Health Conditions

In Chapters 11 through 13, we detail the relationships (positive, negative, and neutral) between hormone therapy (HT) and cardiovascular disease, breast cancer, and other forms of cancer. But, from time to time, you probably read newspaper articles or see a report on the evening news about a number of other health conditions that are supposedly linked to the use of HT. Well, it's time to set the record straight, and that's what we do in this chapter. This chapter reviews a number of conditions you may hear discussed in the same breath as HT. But, in most instances, research hasn't convincingly shown HT to impact these conditions one way or the other.

In this chapter, we define each of these conditions, discuss the signs and symptoms, and review how the conditions have been linked to HT. We discuss the symptoms because, whether they're linked to HT or not, these conditions usually affect folks who are over the age of 40, so you may want to be aware of them.

Dealing with Deep Vein Thrombosis and Other Impeding Issues

Deep vein thrombosis (DVT) is probably not a term you use everyday, and it's probably not a term you want to hear from your doctor. To start with, thrombosis is not a musical instrument with a sliding handle. A *thrombosis* is a five-dollar word for a *blood clot* (a lump of coagulated blood) that forms in a deep vein and impairs the flow of blood through the vein.

How deep do you have to look to find these deep veins? Good question, but don't expect the answer to be as deep as a discussion on the meaning of life. To find deep veins, you have to look no farther than the veins in your upper arms, your legs, and your pelvis, but DVT most commonly occurs in your leg. These veins lie deeper under the skin than surface veins and return more blood to the heart. A clot in one of these veins can cause more complications than a clot in surface veins.

What's so bad about DVT? Another good question. If a clot forms in one of these deep veins and then breaks off, it can flow to the lung. When a clot reaches the lung, it can become lodged and cause a blockage. The blockage is called a *pulmonary embolism* — *pulmonary* meaning it's *in the lungs* and *embolism* meaning *a part of a blood clot*.

A DVT in your upper arm is much less likely to cause problems such as a pulmonary embolism than a DVT in your upper thigh or pelvic region. DVTs in the upper part of the leg cause 95 percent of pulmonary embolisms.

The way the blood gets clotted in the first place is where hormone therapy enters the explanatory picture. Medical types first discovered the hormone/clot association when birth-control pills became available. Women who smoked and took birth-control pills seemed to have a higher incidence of blood clots and *phlebitis* (inflammation of a blood vein). The body of recent research on hormone therapy and blood-clotting conditions, such as DVT and pulmonary embolism, is growing and some patterns are forming.

Recognizing the signs

By far, the most troublesome and common cases of DVT occur in the upper part of the leg, so we want to let you in on ways to recognize a DVT in your leg, though you should keep in mind that only about half of people with DVT in their legs have symptoms. If you do have symptoms, you may notice some of these signs:

- **Pain or tenderness:** Symptoms may occur in your calf or thigh, sometimes only when standing or walking.
- **Redness:** Your leg may look red as though you bumped it.
- **Swelling:** Your entire leg may swell, or the swelling may be confined to a blood vessel, which creates a ridge of swelling that you can feel.
- **Warmth:** Your leg may feel warm to the touch.

And here's how you can recognize a blood clot in your lung (pulmonary embolism):

- Chest pain that gets worse with a deep breath
- Cough that may bring up blood
- Sudden shortness of breath

Your thigh is the most likely location for a blood clot — at least the first time you get one. Clots like these are likely to cause considerable pain — enough pain that most people call their doctor or go to the hospital. That's a good instinct to follow because these clots need to be treated before they do major damage to nearby tissues or break off and travel toward the lungs.

Sometimes, your leg can become bluish because the blood is having a hard time getting back to the heart. The blood is blue and not red because it no longer contains oxygen. After blood delivers its oxygen to other parts of the body, it returns to the lungs for an oxygen refill.

Determining the role of hormones

Studies in the mid-1990s flip-flopped on the hormone issue. Some research indicated that women on estrogen therapy were more likely to have blood clots in the legs, *phlebitis* (inflammation of the veins), and *pulmonary embolus* (blood clots in the lung). Other studies showed no clotting-related effects at all. Now that's a lot of help, isn't it?

But a growing body of evidence exists, culminating in the well-organized Women's Health Initiative (WHI) study, that shows a correlation between the use of conjugated estrogen therapy and blood-clotting problems. A variety of studies, including the WHI, found that the risk of DVT or pulmonary embolism doubles for women who use conjugated equine estrogen. The risk is greatest during the first year of use.

Determining the reason behind the clotting connection is more controversial. Some medical and research groups believe that *not all forms of estrogen* would have this effect on women. They believe that the *type* of estrogen (conjugated estrogen) is responsible for the increase in clotting. Conjugated equine estrogens, such as those tested by the WHI, are known to be a more potent form of estrogen than estrogens found naturally in a human body, which may cause unwanted affects. Research in the future may show that hormone therapy using natural estradiol (which the body uses more easily than conjugated equine estrogen) won't increase the risk of DVT or pulmonary embolism. But, to date, only conjugated equine estrogen has been thoroughly tested, and the results indicate an increase in DVT and pulmonary embolism with use during the first year.

Some medical thoroughbreds also question whether it was the conjugated estrogen or the use of progesterin that raised the risk of clotting; estrogen alone didn't seem to increase the clotting risk as significantly. These folks suggest that using combined estrogen and progesterin may be more risky.

The hormone-delivery method may also make a difference to your risk of developing clotting problems such as DVT or pulmonary embolism. The WHI study tested only an oral form of estrogen, and many women administer hormone therapy through a skin patch. Some doctors and researchers suggest that conclusions can't be drawn about the skin patch because researchers only tested an oral form of the hormone. Medical folks know that the body processes the estrogen from a patch differently than estrogen from a pill. (Pills are processed by the liver before being distributed to the bloodstream; patches bypass the liver-processing step. For more information on all the different forms of estrogen and delivery methods, turn to Chapter 10.)

The skin-patch delivery method hasn't been linked to higher incidence of blood-clotting problems or phlebitis. However, it will take more research to discover whether estradiol skin patches are less harmful than conjugated-estrogen pills. In the meantime, carefully consider the risk of DVT and other blood-clotting problems, particularly when using conjugated-estrogen pills in hormone therapy.

 Women with a history of blood-clotting problems should approach hormone use cautiously. A hormone therapy regimen consisting of the estradiol form of estrogen delivered through a patch is probably the safest bet for most women.

Dissecting Diabetes

Diabetes is a huge health problem in the United States. *Diabetes* is characterized by high levels of *glucose* (sugar) in the blood. These high glucose levels are the result of the body's inability to absorb the sugar a person eats.

 Insulin is a hormone that acts as the great facilitator in the blood-to-tissue glucose-transfer process. When the glucose levels in your blood get relatively high, your pancreas releases insulin to help your cells absorb the sugar in your blood and use it for energy. When the pancreas doesn't produce enough (or produces no) insulin, diabetes is the result.

Two basic reasons explain why some people can't transfer glucose from their blood to their tissue:

- Their body can't make enough insulin.
- The tissues quit responding to insulin and won't take in glucose.

Several kinds of diabetes exist:

- **Type-1 diabetes:** No one knows what causes type-1 diabetes, but the condition is genetic. (It was once called *juvenile-onset diabetes* because the majority of sufferers are diagnosed before their 20th birthday.)
- **Type-2 diabetes:** This form of diabetes is the most common form and is most often diagnosed in people over 40 years of age. Eighty percent of people with this form of diabetes are overweight. Excess weight in combination with age triggers type-2 diabetes.

Recognizing the signs

Nearly 16 million people in the United States and over 2 million people in Canada live with diabetes. The American Diabetes Association says another 5 million Americans are walking around with the disease but don't know it. If three or four of these symptoms describe your state of affairs, and they persist for more than a month, get the situation checked out.

- Extreme thirst (causing you to drink an unusual amount of fluids)
- Frequent urination
- Constant hunger
- Unexpected weight loss
- Fatigue
- Itchy skin or genitals
- Pain or numbness in your extremities
- Slow-healing wounds

Determining the role of hormones

No one has yet demonstrated that hormone therapy actually leads to diabetes. Some very small and short-term studies suggest that hormone therapy could slightly increase your blood-glucose levels. Don't worry about it. Most other studies found absolutely no increase in risk of diabetes for women who take HT. The WHI study results published in 2002 didn't even mention this side effect, so raising your glucose level shouldn't be a big concern if you're using hormone therapy.

Facing the Facts about Fibromyalgia

Ever heard of this one? Well, nearly 80 percent of the people who suffer from fibromyalgia are women, and most of them are over 40 years of age. The laundry list of symptoms may make you say, "You've gotta be kidding," but we're not fibbing about fibromyalgia.

Fibromyalgia is a chronic condition in which you experience widespread muscle and soft-tissue pain, tenderness, and fatigue. You may experience pain in up to 18 specific areas that are aptly named *tender points* or *trigger points* (many of which are clustered around your neck).

Fibromyalgia is normally first diagnosed in women between the ages of 30 and 50, but we also know a few women who were first diagnosed in their seventies.

Recognizing the signs

Fibromyalgia symptoms are very general but intense. They include

- Stiffness and soreness, especially in the morning.
- Extremely tender places on your body, especially where tendons and muscles meet (on the inside of your elbows and in your hips and knees, for example). Pain in 11 of the 18 tender points is usually the threshold doctors look for in diagnosing this condition.
- Difficulty getting a full night's sleep.
- General fatigue.
- Irritability, mood changes, and depression.
- Problems with eye muscles. (Your eye may turn inward or close slightly.)
- Numbness, burning, or cold sensations in your hands and feet.

Some people with fibromyalgia also experience less common problems with their memory or concentration, have difficulty hearing or can't tolerate some sounds, and suffer migraine headaches.

If you suffer from fibromyalgia, or suspect that you do, you may want to check out *Fibromyalgia For Dummies* (Roland Staud with Christine Adamec, Wiley Publishing, Inc.) in addition to reading the following "Determining the role of hormones" section.

Determining the role of hormones

The cause of fibromyalgia isn't well understood. Most scientists believe that some type of hormonal imbalance causes the condition, but they can't agree on which hormones are unbalanced. Given the symptoms, researchers are focusing their suspicions on these areas:

- Brain chemicals that control mood and can also cause a disrupted sleep cycle
- Hormones released by the pituitary gland (which are also found in the brain and are sensitive to estrogen)
- Deficiencies in growth hormones

A link to the female sex hormones also seems likely because fibromyalgia is most likely to occur

- In women approaching menopause or who have gone through menopause
- In women who have just had a baby (especially women over 35)
- A few years after women have had a tubal ligation or a hysterectomy

Getting the Goods on Gallbladder Disease

The gallbladder is a warehouse for *bile,* a greenish liquid that helps digest fats. The gallbladder is supposed to take the bile from the liver and inject it into the intestines (where it goes to work) via a bile duct. When too much cholesterol is present in the bile, the cholesterol hardens, forming crystals inside the gallbladder. The crystals then come together to form *gallstones.*

Recognizing the signs

Most people don't even know they have gallstones. They experience no symptoms and only find the stones when they're tested for some other condition (like ulcers or kidney stones). Any pain is usually like a dull ache or cramping. But large or numerous gallstones can cause noticeable pain, vomiting, or nausea. The pain comes on fast and strong and lasts from 30 minutes to several hours. You feel it in your upper abdomen under your ribcage. Sometimes the pain radiates, moving all the way through your lower back or up to your right shoulder. Some people become nauseous and feverish.

If you have a high fever or chills, your *bile duct* (pathway to the small intestine) may be inflamed or blocked. A blocked bile duct can also cause urine to be dark yellow, stool to be light in color, and skin to take on a yellow cast. The symptoms often occur at night or after eating (especially a high-fat meal).

If gallstones cause other infections, doctors usually remove your gallbladder, but gallstones themselves are rarely a life-threatening condition.

Determining the role of hormones

Estrogen has been tagged as a promoter of gallstones. One of the most commonly prescribed estrogens in hormone therapy is conjugated estrogen in pill form. Because the pill has to be digested in the liver before entering the bloodstream, it tends to increases the level of LDL cholesterol (the bad stuff) in the bile. Raising the level of cholesterol in the bile can increase the risk of gallstone formation.

You may be able to avoid gallbladder issues altogether by using estrogen in patch form instead of taking pills. The patch avoids an estrogen trip through the liver, so you don't risk adding more cholesterol to the gallbladder and increasing the chances of gallstone formation.

Looking at Lupus

Lupus is the short name for a disease called *systemic lupus erythematosus*. Although lupus is a fairly rare disease, it's much more common among women than men — particularly women between the ages of 15 and 45.

Because lupus is a disease of the immune system, it attacks nearly every organ in your body. The immune system normally protects your body from infections. However, with lupus, the immune system starts attacking "friendly" tissues in your own body. This creates havoc in your body, causing tissue damage and illness.

Lupus is a complex disease, and researchers have yet to determine the cause. The likely scenario is that no single cause exists. Instead, a combination of genetic, environmental, and possibly hormonal factors may work together to cause the disease.

The hormone connection is curious. If you look at the U.S. population in general, only one out of 2,000 people have lupus. But, if you only consider women between the ages of 14 and 45 years old, one in 250 have the disease. This leads scientists to conclude that the female sex hormones are somehow involved in this disease.

Recognizing the signs

Lupus can affect many parts of the body, and it often attacks the joints, skin, kidneys, heart, lungs, blood vessels, and brain. Although people with the disease may have many different symptoms, some of the most common symptoms are

✔ Extreme fatigue

✔ Kidney problems

✔ Painful, swollen, inflamed joints (arthritis)

✔ Skin rashes and inflammation

✔ Unexplained fever

Many women who have lupus initially think that their swollen or stiff joints are simply caused by arthritis. In fact, some researchers believe that lupus is related to rheumatoid arthritis. If left untreated, lupus can cause many complications.

Determining the role of hormones

Given that women of childbearing age are at greatest risk of this disease, it's not surprising that researchers have found an increase in lupus among women taking hormone therapy. The specifics are not understood, but the correlation between female hormones (including those taken as hormone therapy) and lupus looks suspicious.

One particularly large study found that women who were taking hormone therapy had double the risk of developing lupus compared with menopausal women not taking hormone therapy. The longer women used estrogen, the greater their risk of developing the disease. No one knows the reason for these results.

If you have a family history of lupus, you may want to consider an alternative to hormone therapy for your perimenopausal and menopausal symptoms (check out Chapter 17 for some alternatives).

Monitoring Migraines

The cause of migraines isn't known for certain, but roughly 10 to 11 percent of people in the United States and Canada suffer from them, and most migraine sufferers are women. Most women who have migraines are between the ages of 30 and 49 and have a family history of migraines.

For years, scientists thought that migraine headaches occurred when the blood vessels in the brain suddenly constricted (got smaller) and then expanded. More recently, researchers are suggesting that migraines are caused by inherited abnormalities in certain areas of the brain.

Recognizing the signs

Migraine headaches are like everyday headaches, but they're a whole lot worse. They're more intense, they throb, they often affect only one side of the head, and they're often accompanied by nausea, vomiting, and sensitivity to light and/or noise. Some people also see *auras,* which are flashing lights or blind spots in their field of vision.

Determining the role of hormones

Many factors can trigger a migraine attack, and fluctuations in estrogen levels may be one of them. A sudden drop in estrogen encourages a migraine in women who are predisposed to them. Medical folks don't understand the hormone connection real well, particularly in light of the new thoughts on what causes migraines, but it's very suspicious that

✔ Seventy percent of migraine sufferers are women.

✔ Women who have migraines during their menstrual cycles generally report them during the part of the cycle when estrogen levels drop.

✔ Women often report that migraines go away during pregnancy.

Many women first suffer these headaches during their reproductive years, specifically a day or two before their period or the first day or two of their period when estrogen levels drop. Other women get migraines around the time they ovulate, when estrogen levels again drop.

Migraines seem to happen when estrogen drops, so the fact that many women experience migraines in response to menopause isn't too surprising.

The active form of estrogen in HT relieves the symptoms associated with migraines. Women on a cyclical hormone therapy regimen (one in which you quit taking estrogen for a few days each month) are more likely to have migraines because of rapid drops in estrogen. Continuous hormone therapy may prevent the headaches.

Chapter 15

Making the Decision about Hormone Therapy

*W*e want to start this chapter by encouraging you to return to it periodically over the next few years. Your decisions about coping with perimenopause and menopause will probably change as your health changes, your priorities shift, and new options become available. This evaluation process doesn't end with a one-time pronouncement that you have to follow for the rest of your life. You can (and should!) revisit your alternatives periodically.

Outlining Attitudes about HT

Most women going through the change fall into one of three camps when it comes to hormone therapy (HT).

✔ "Natural is beautiful. If we were meant to have estrogen all our lives, we would have been born that way."

✔ "There's no way I want to live a day without my hormones!"

✔ "I've tried hormones, and they were awful. I guess I'll just have to put up with the symptoms."

Over time, you may move from one camp to the next — and then back again. If your symptoms interfere with the quality of your life during perimenopause, you may want to take hormones for a few years to ease the transition into menopause and then taper off medication as your symptoms decrease.

Updating HT recommendations

The results from the Women's Health Initiative (WHI) study released in 2002 seemed to put the kibosh on hormone therapy (HT). The study evaluated the use of a combination estrogen and progestin as a means of lowering the risk of cardiovascular disease in women. After several years, the answer became clear. Not only did this combination of hormones *not* lower the risk of cardiovascular disease, it actually increased the risk of breast cancer, heart attacks, strokes, and blood clots. Based on these findings, the National Institutes of Health, the sponsor of the study, terminated the trial several years ahead of schedule.

But the WHI findings are neither surprising nor applicable to all forms of HT. The study evaluated the use of a specific HT product (conjugated equine estrogen plus MPA progestin). This specific estrogen product, derived from female horse urine, is one of the most commonly prescribed forms, but one that was already known to have problems. Other major studies performed in the 1980s and 1990s showed that horse-derived estrogens may produce higher risks of heart disease than the natural estradiol form of estrogen.

The specific HT product administered in the test uses MPA (medroxyprogesterone acetate) as the progestin part of the therapy; this also wasn't the best choice. Researchers have known for more than ten years that MPA causes more blood vessel damage and reverses more of the positive effects of estrogen than natural progesterone.

In essence, the WHI study simply confirms the information that we've known for about 20 years — the most-prescribed HT product is not a good choice for menopausal women.

To be fair, the WHI study is one of the biggest, best organized, and best controlled studies of HT and its effects on women's health ever conducted. If you want to know how conjugated estrogen and MPA affect women after menopause, the WHI has some hard facts on the benefits and risks. But, the study leads us to wonder if *all* HT regimens would have the same results. We know that pills have different effects than patches, and we know that conjugated estrogen has different effects than estradiol estrogen. We don't know if these other HT regimens have the same health risks as the one tested in the WHI study.

The purpose of HT is to bring your hormones into a "healthy" balance. The "natural is beautiful" group argues that what's normal at 25 isn't normal at 55, and they're correct. Unfortunately, the low levels of estrogen that are "normal" at 55 often result in physical and mental discomfort.

The problem is that your body doesn't produce a substitute for estrogen when your ovaries quit producing the hormone. When your body stops getting the estrogen it's used to having, it lets you know with messages in the form of hot flashes, memory lapses, vaginal dryness, bone loss, and shifting blood cholesterol levels, all of which are typical of sustained, low levels of estrogen

If you have a family or personal history that includes osteoporosis or colorectal cancer, HT may be the right choice for you. Keep in mind that other medications can be helpful too. (Check out Chapter 17 for information on treating osteoporosis without hormones.)

Taking hormone therapy does present health risks. Estrogen encourages the growth of some breast cancers and may also be a problem for women with gall-bladder or liver problems, blood clots, or undiagnosed vaginal bleeding. So how do you decide? Business people often perform cost-benefit analyses, a very rational approach in which you list the benefits and the costs (in this case risks) and make a logical decision. The information in this chapter (and other HT-related chapters in this book) can help you perform a cost-benefit analysis.

As with any personal decision, you also have to consider your values, lifestyle preferences, and personal prejudices and preferences — illogical as some of them may be. Also, look at your medical history and that of your family. You may eventually face the same medical problems that affect your parents, siblings, or grandparents. We help you sort through these issues, too.

Weighing the Benefits and Risks of HT

Most women consider hormone therapy (HT) only because their symptoms are making their lives miserable, which is also known as "negatively affecting your quality of life." Only you can determine if your quality of life is at risk. (Check out the "Figuring out just how bad it really is" sidebar to get an objective look at your symptoms.)

Realizing the benefits

HT relieves perimenopausal and menopausal symptoms and protects your body against a variety of serious medical conditions. You can find information about these benefits throughout this book (Chapter 10 is a good place to start), but we put them all together here so you can do a quick side-by-side comparison as you're trying to make your decision. HT relieves

- Bone deterioration
- Fuzzy thinking
- Hot flashes
- Insomnia and fitful sleep due to hot flashes or night sweats
- Memory lapses
- Vaginal dryness and *atrophy* (thinning and shrinking)

Some evidence points to the fact that the mental and emotional symptoms are actually worse during perimenopause than after you're officially menopausal. The wild hormone fluctuations are probably the culprit.

If you're experiencing many of the perimenopausal symptoms described in the "Figuring out just how bad it really is" sidebar, but they appear at about the same time each month — prior to your period — and then go away for some length of time during each menstrual cycle, you probably have pre-menstrual syndrome rather than perimenopausal symptoms.

By raising the level of estrogen in your body during the latter 20 to 40 years of your life, you can protect yourself against a number of disabling conditions:

- ✔ Cardiovascular disease, which includes arteriosclerosis, heart attack, and heart disease
- ✔ Colon cancer
- ✔ Elevated LDL ("bad" cholesterol) and *triglyceride* (another bad cholesterol) levels
- ✔ Osteoporosis (weakening of the bones)

You may be the type of woman who marches through perimenopause, refusing to let those annoying symptoms interfere with your life. Maybe getting relief from the symptoms just didn't seem to be worth the risks that HT may contribute to other health problems. Or maybe you barely experienced any symptoms.

As you approach menopause, the risks and rewards of HT may look different to you. The statistics, which we put on paper in the following sections, are fairly dramatic. The decision scales may become more balanced; you may even throw up your hands and say, "Damned if I do, damned if I don't." What can you do to sort through the decision-making process? Read on. While you're reading, take your family medical history and personal health concerns into account. And keep in mind that you can always take a fresh look at the situation next month or next year.

Helping your heart stay healthy

Out of a group of 100 women who are 50 years old, 20 of them will develop heart disease before their 80th birthday. But, if you put all 100 women on hormones, only 10 will develop heart disease before they turn 80. Figure 15-1 provides a graphic representation.

Pretty impressive, but here's the caveat: During the first and second years of hormone use, the risk of heart disease is actually greater than it is without hormones. After the second year, researchers are divided on the benefits of hormone therapy. A very large and frequently mentioned study, the Nurses' Health Study, found the risk of heart disease decreases after the second year of hormone use, and over time, the use of estrogen cuts the risk of heart disease in half.

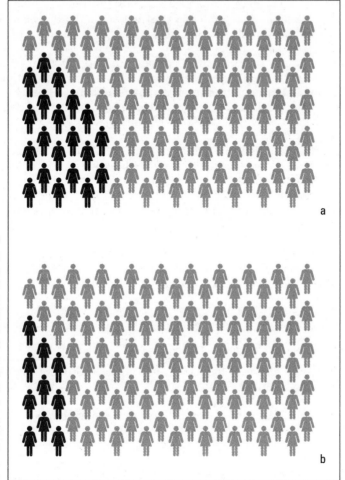

Figure 15-1:
Twenty of a
hundred
50-year-old
women will
develop
heart
disease
before
they're 80
(a). If they
all take HT,
that number
is cut in
half (b).

The Nurses' Health Study isn't the only study that showed women using hormone therapy had a lower risk of heart disease. So many people were surprised when the Women's Health Initiative (WHI) study recently concluded that hormone therapy actually increases the risk of heart disease with extended use. Why did the WHI findings differ so radically from prior studies? Did the specific type of combination therapy (Prempro) the WHI participants used cause the results? The medical community hasn't formulated an answer to those questions quite yet, but researchers are fast at work to see if other types of hormones yield the same result.

The WHI results have already caused two women doctors to head back to the books to reevaluate the old studies. What did they find during their reexamination? A group of women with similar lifestyles (they exercise, they don't drink a lot of alcohol, and they eat a healthy diet) had less heart disease than other women whether or not they took hormones.

At this point in time, it appears that hormone therapy shouldn't be the first line of defense in treating or preventing heart disease or heart attack. And you should avoid hormone therapy if you have a history of heart disease or heart attack. The first line of defense against heart disease and heart attack should be a healthy diet, regular exercise, and an overall healthy lifestyle.

It's important to note that researchers stopped the WHI study, but they didn't put the brakes on because participants were in grave danger of dying from a heart attack or heart disease. (Although use of hormone therapy seemed to increase the risk of heart attack, it didn't increase the risk of dying from a heart attack.) Researchers halted the study because of the increased risk in breast cancer.

What about other types of cardiovascular disease such as fatty blood (high LDL and triglyceride levels) and *hypertension* (high blood pressure)? Glad you asked. Estrogen is a mixed bag as far as cholesterol and triglycerides are concerned:

- ✔ Estrogen lowers LDL levels (by as much as 15 percent in one study).
- ✔ Some forms of estrogen raise HDL ("good" cholesterol) levels.
- ✔ Oral estrogen seems to increase triglycerides (boo), but the patch tends to lower triglycerides (yeah).

The moral of this story is that if you have a problem with blood cholesterol and triglycerides, you need to find the right type of estrogen to keep them in check.

Estrogen's benefits are clearer in relation to high blood pressure. It helps dilate blood vessels and improve blood flow, both of which lower your blood pressure.

The jury is still out on the impact of estrogen on stroke. High doses of estrogen seem to increase the risk of stroke slightly in menopausal women. This shouldn't be a problem anymore because today's HT regimens use low-dosage estrogen. Still, research confirms a slight increase in the risk of stroke during the first two years of use. After the first two years, estrogen actually seems to lower the risk of stroke in women taking HT.

Lifting the veil on combination HT and your heart

Now, when you add *progestin* (synthetic forms of the hormone progesterone) to the hormone therapy, everything changes. Progestins seem to dull the positive effects of estrogen on your cardiovascular system. Here are the findings for HT containing estrogen and progestin:

- ✔ It lowers HDL cholesterol (when taken in pill form).
- ✔ It raises triglycerides (when taken in pill form).

Unfortunately, if you have a uterus and want to take HT, the progestin must be included. But a variety of progestins are available, and patches have less of a negative impact on cholesterol than pills. Natural progesterone, ground up so your body can absorb it, doesn't seem to dull the effects of estrogen as much as progestins.

Before the WHI study, most doctors agreed that women could lower their risk of cardiovascular problems by using HT. Most doctors now agree that combination HT shouldn't be the first line of defense against cardiovascular disease.

Here's the $64-million question: Could it be that conjugated estrogen and MPA progestin (the hormone therapy tested in the WHI study) produce more hazardous side effects than other, more natural, forms of hormone therapy (estradiol and natural progesterone, for example)? Well, we all have to stay tuned for the answer to that question. It's not really appropriate to take the results of the WHI study and say that all combination hormone therapy regimens would create the same hazards to your cardiovascular system. But just so you know, here's what the WHI study concluded regarding the Prempro combination HT regimen:

- ✔ The risk of stroke doesn't increase during the first year of HT use, but it increases over time — after the first year for about five years (even in healthy women).
- ✔ Your risk of suffering a heart attack increases while taking HT, *but* you're not more likely to die of a heart attack while taking HT compared to women who don't take HT at all.

Avoiding bone breaks

HT dramatically reduces the risk of osteoporosis and the debilitating results of the disease in Caucasian and Asian women (check out Figure 15-2). The top figure (a) shows the number of women out of 100 who will suffer a hip fracture after age 50 — 15. The next figure (b) shows the number of hip fractures in women 50 or older who take hormone therapy — 11. Because African-American women have a lower incidence of osteoporosis, use of HT only slightly lowers their risk of fracture.

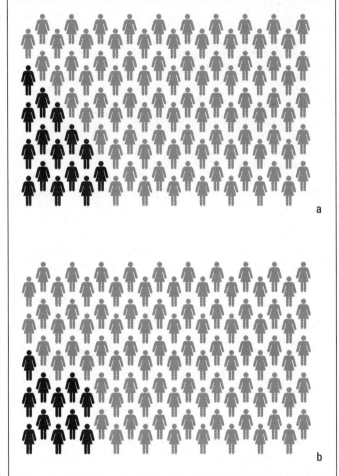

Figure 15-2:
Risk of hip
fracture in
women 50
and older
(a) without
and (b) with
hormones.

Most women lose about 3 percent of bone mass each year after menopause. Postmenopausal women who take HT regularly for ten years don't lose bone mass; they actually increase their bone mass by about 6 percent!

Because women on HT regimens lose less bone (or even build bone) during menopause, they also have a lower incidence of hip fractures. HT users are about 25 percent less likely to fracture a hip. That stat is pretty significant, particularly when you consider how debilitating hip fractures are to women after menopause. (Many women require care for the rest of their life after suffering a broken hip.)

The protective effects of HT on your bone only last as long as you take hormones. So when you stop — wham — you begin losing bone mass quickly.

Keeping colon cancer at bay

Here's another one of those "we don't know exactly why, but it does" benefits of HT. While you take HT, you have a slightly lower risk of developing colon cancer. After you discontinue using hormones, the protection gradually disappears.

Considering the risks

HT also presents some risks to women:

- ✔ **Increases your risk of endometrial cancer if you take estrogen without also taking progesterone.** Today, doctors no longer prescribe estrogen without balancing it with progesterone, so this isn't much of a problem anymore. Unless you've had a hysterectomy, your doctor won't prescribe estrogen alone (see Chapter 13).

- ✔ **Increases your risk of gallbladder problems.** Although we have the statistics to prove that HT increases your risk of gallstones (particularly when taken in pill form for more than five years), researchers don't know the particulars concerning why this is the case (see Chapter 14). The risk can be lowered by using a patch instead of a pill.

- ✔ **May increase your risk of breast cancer.** Some breast cancers, but not all breast cancers, depend on estrogen to grow. Because HT raises estrogen levels, taking it may encourage estrogen-related breast cancer. The evidence is stacking up on this issue (see Chapter 12).

- ✔ **May increase your risk of deep-vein blood clots.** If you experienced clotting during a pregnancy or while using birth-control pills, you may have a problem with HT as well, particularly if you smoke. Chapter 14 talks about the relationship between clots and HT.

- ✔ **May increase your risk of heart attack and coronary heart disease.** The scales are starting to tip in the direction that HT may actually increase your risk of heart problems rather than lower it. The jury is still out: This finding may be less true of HT that uses skin patches as the method of delivery and estradiol as the estrogen, as opposed to other forms of HT.

Having trouble deciding if you're at risk for osteoporosis, cardiovascular disease, or breast cancer? We have three little quizzes to help you look objectively at your risk factors in Figures 15-3, 15-4, and 15-5. The lists are a very simple first step to assess your risks — high, low, or in between. You can't predict your chances of getting a particular disease based on your answers, but the more statements you agree with, the greater your risk for that condition.

Osteoporosis Risk Sheet

1. My mother and/or sister has osteoporosis.
2. I am "small-boned".
3. I am Caucasian or Asian.
4. I am older than 65 years of age.
5. I have breast fed my child/children for at least three months.
6. I have lost at least an inch in height.
7. I have taken cortisone or corticosteroids for over five years.
8. My periods stopped before I was forty.
9. My ovaries were removed before I was forty.
10. I get less than 1,200 mg of calcium each day.
11. I exercise less than an $1^1/2$ hours a week.
12. I smoke.
13. I was anorexic for a period in my life.
14. I drink 3 or more cups of coffee a day (or the equivalent amount of caffeine as found in colas, chocolate, and so on).

You are in a higher risk category for osteoporosis if you agree with questions 1–4.

Figure 15-3:
Evaluating your risk for osteoporosis.

Heart Disease Risk Sheet

1. My mother had a heart attack before she was 65 years old/my dad had a heart attack before 55 years of age.
2. I have had a heart attack.
3. I have hypertension (high blood pressure).
4. My HDL cholesterol is less than 50.
5. My Cholesterol to HDL ratio is over 3.0.
6. My triglycerides are over 120.
7. I have diabetes.
8. I have chest pain (angina) or heart flutters (fibrillation) on occasion.
9. I typically eat more than 50 grams of fat a day.
10. I smoke.
11. I'm overweight.
12. I exercise less than three times a week or for less than an hour and a half a week.

Figure 15-4:
Evaluating your risk for heart disease.

Breast Cancer Risk Sheet

1. I have had breast cancer.
2. My mother or sister has had breast cancer.
3. My grandmothers had breast cancer.
4. There is colon, endometrial, ovarian, or cervical cancer in my family.
5. I gave birth to my first child after age 35.
6. I am over 35 and have never had a baby.
7. I have at least three alcoholic drinks a week.

Agreeing with the first three statements puts you in a fairly high risk category.

Figure 15-5:
Evaluating
your risk
for breast
cancer.

It's important to realize that *risk* is not the same as *certainty*. We all know people who smoked and drank and lived a long life and others who lived healthy and exercised and died of a heart attack well before their time. But, in between these unlikely extremes, you can evaluate your risk factors and try to take some steps to improve your chances of preventing disease.

Many women choose to weigh their risk of osteoporosis and cardiovascular disease against their risk of breast cancer because HT protects you from osteoporosis but may raise your risk for breast cancer, and depending on what form of HT you take, it may or may not help protect you from heart disease.

If you are at great risk of osteoporosis or cardiovascular disease but have few risk factors for breast cancer, HT may be for you. If you're at great risk for breast cancer, you may want to consider other alternatives for protecting your bones and heart. Chapters 16 through 19 give you some great ideas about alternatives.

Some of the risk factors for each of the conditions are things that you can control by modifying your lifestyle, eating preferences, or other behaviors. You can lower these risks immediately by making some changes.

Some studies indicate that use of HT slightly increases your risk of breast cancer (other studies show no effect whatsoever — so it's still controversial). If you're worried about your risk of breast cancer, take an objective look at your personal risk factors for the disease.

Summing Up the Studies

If you've made it this far through the chapter, you've digested a lot of information, and your plate is probably still full. We thought we'd included a little synopsis at this point to help you separate your peas from your potatoes, regroup, re-energize, and re-weigh the risks and benefits associated with hormone therapy.

You should realize that the best-studied type of HT is the regimen in which women take a daily pill that contains both conjugated equine estrogen and MPA progestin. Studies of other regimens are more scattered in terms of the size of the study group and the types of HT investigated. So these results are heavily biased toward the benefits and risks of combination therapy using conjugated estrogen and MPA progestin. (For more information on all the different types of therapies and hormones, check out Chapter 10.) For now, Tables 15-1 and 15-2 provide a summary of the short- and long-term benefits and risks of HT.

Table 15-1 Just the Facts Ma'am: HT Benefits during Use	
Short-Term Use (Less Than 5 Years)	**Long-Term Use (5 Years or More)**
Improved mental skills (verbal memory and reasoning)	Increased bone density
Improved sense of well-being	Reduction of hip fractures
Decrease in sleep interruption	Reduction of spinal fractures
Decrease in *urogenital atrophy* (atrophy of the vagina and urinary tract)	Reduction of colon cancer
Decrease in mood swings	Decrease in dementia
Decrease in hot flashes	

Table 15-2 Just the Facts Ma'am, Part II: HT Risks during Use	
Short-Term Use (Less Than 5 Years)	**Long-Term Use (5 Years or More)**
Possible increase in breast cancer	Increase in breast cancer
Increase in gallbladder disease	Significant increase in gallbladder disease
Increase in heart attack	Slight increase in heart attack
Slight increase in stroke	Slight increase in stroke
Significant increase in deep-vein clots	Increase in deep-vein clots

Studying the studies: What you need to know before you panic over news stories

Conflicting reports on the risks and benefits associated with HT make the decision about taking HT really confusing. Magazines, newspapers, and talking heads on TV constantly present you with new studies proving that everything you've read in the past is wrong. This cuts both ways. One week someone says that the risks of HT have been blown way out of proportion. The next week you read that HT does absolutely nothing to help menopausal women. (See the "Updating HT recommendations" sidebar in this chapter.)

One reason opinions swing so far in each direction has nothing whatsoever to do with HT, itself, but has everything to do with how the studies are conducted. Without getting too complicated, experts basically conduct three types of studies: descriptive, observational, and controlled trials.

Descriptive studies simply describe what happened to patients or groups of people. For example, one doctor may report that all her patients who experienced hot flashes had blue eyes. From this information, you can't really say that blue eyes cause hot flashes, but such a report may be interesting to experts studying hot flashes (or experts studying people with blue eyes).

Observational studies observe people in the settings of their everyday lives. Researchers interview study participants over an extended period of time about their lifestyles, medical histories, existing medical conditions, and medications. A good thing about observational studies is that you can find a good-size group of people who have been taking a medication or participating in a therapy over a long period of time. The disadvantage is that no real *control* is in place. Participants do whatever they want and don't have to limit themselves to one particular therapy. You can detect patterns, but you can only speculate about what caused those patterns.

In *controlled trials,* participants are generally separated into two groups — one that uses the therapy being studied and a *control group* that takes a *placebo* (form of therapy that outwardly resembles the therapy being tested but provides no medicinal or curative properties) or nothing at all. In these kinds of studies, researchers can determine the cause if a change occurs. The best controlled trials are *randomized,* meaning that researchers randomly assign people to a therapy group. Comparisons of the groups can be objective, without the chance that the person sorting the participants accidentally put all the sick people in one group and all the healthy people in the other, for example.

Basically, each type of study has merits and drawbacks. Descriptive and observational studies can shed light on patterns of disease or medical conditions, but they can't demonstrate the exact *cause* of a particular effect. You can show that some kind of link exists between certain factors and a particular disease or condition, but you can't really describe the details of the link. Controlled studies are designed to determine causes. That doesn't mean that controlled trials are the only valuable studies, though many experts insist that controlled, randomized trials are the only way to go when making medical recommendations.

The next time you see an alarming headline in your favorite magazine or newspaper that casts doubt on everything you've ever read about menopause or HT, read the details. Make sure that the conclusions drawn from the study (and the resulting claims) don't reach further than the study method permits. But also make sure that researchers and writers aren't throwing the baby out with the bathwater by dismissing studies simply because they aren't randomized, controlled trials.

Presenting the Options for Perimenopause

In the following sections, we present several ways that women deal with peri-menopausal symptoms. Even though we group them into individual options, you may want to mix and match. For example, we discuss diet and exercise, herbal solutions, and HT in separate sections. But adopting better eating and exercise habits can only enhance the positive aspects of herbs or HT.

Option 1: The lifestyle solution

If you're perimenopausal and your symptoms annoy you but rarely interfere with your life, you may want to make some lifestyle changes to alleviate them. (Chapters 18 and 19 can help you renew your commitment to keeping your body fit and healthy in this new season of your life.) Many women find that some of the symptoms of perimenopause fade with a renewed focus on getting or staying fit.

Some of the anxiety and irritability you're experiencing probably stems from feeling out of control about the changes going on with your body. Adding a couple pounds a year and losing muscle tone isn't unusual for perimenopausal women, but it's also not caused by changes in your hormones. As people move into their forties and fifties, they often devote less time to their personal needs than they devote to the demands of their families and careers. A healthy diet and exercise plan can put you in control of your body and improve your state of mind.

Regular physical activity improves mental functions such as memory, con-centration, self-confidence, and self-esteem. It also reduces stress, which can trigger hot flashes, interrupted sleep, and irritability. But it's not all mental. Only about one in 20 women who exercise regularly report experiencing hot flashes, compared to one out of four less-active women.

Eating a healthy diet, as described in Chapter 18, will boost your immune system, help maintain bone density, and keep your blood lean so you lower your risk of cardiovascular disease and reverse some of the effects of low estrogen levels that define menopause.

Incorporating soy into your diet helps lower your cholesterol, boost your immune system, and prevent hot flashes, and it may lower your risk of breast cancer. (Check out Chapter 16 for more on soy.)

Option 2: The herbal solution

For most women, perimenopausal symptoms are not life threatening so using drugs and hormones to relieve symptoms may seem like using a shotgun to kill mosquitoes.

You may want to consider some non-HT alternatives to alleviate your symptoms. These alternatives can be as diverse as herbs, relaxation techniques, and vaginal lubricants. Herbs of interest for relieving perimenopausal symptoms include black cohosh, soy, dong quai, and ginseng. We cover herbal solutions in detail in Chapter 16.

Stress often triggers hot flashes and anxiety or irritability, so now is a great time to practice relaxation techniques regularly. Don't worry: You don't need to go to Nepal to find a guru. Just take a few minutes each day to do an activity you enjoy, practice some breathing techniques, and give someone a hug. *Biofeedback techniques* (psychological therapy in which you use your mind to control certain body functions) can help you take charge of your breathing and heart rate and lessen your reactions to stressful events or situations. Find out what works for you to reduce the stress in your life — maybe it's yoga, walking, music, or a weekly massage. Chapter 16 explores alternative options.

Option 3: The HT solution

Maybe you aren't wild about taking medication, but your symptoms are interfering with your quality of life; HT may be the answer. HT has been shown to relieve hot flashes because estrogen helps regulate body temperature. In addition, estrogen improves sleep and lowers anxiety by increasing the production and extending the action of *serotonin* (a brain chemical that regulates moods and activity level). Serotonin boosts concentration, improves pain tolerance, enhances memory, and regulates adrenaline so you avoid heart palpitations. Progesterone has been added to the HT regimen to reduce the risk of endometrial cancer that estrogen-only HT would present.

Many women choose to take HT to get rid of their annoying perimenopausal symptoms and may get added protection for their bones and hearts.

If you decide that HT is for you, you still have the option of not using the therapy later on. After a few years, perimenopausal symptoms subside (they don't last forever), and you may decide to limit your use of HT to perimenopause.

The HT option is almost required for women who have their ovaries removed before menopause. Often HT is prescribed prior to surgery or immediately thereafter. Removal of your ovaries is quite a shock to your body because hormone production abruptly ceases. HT can help absorb the shock by replacing the hormones and smoothing things over so you don't experience intense menopausal symptoms, bone loss, or changes in your blood cholesterol.

Remember that many types of estrogen and progesterone are available in many different combinations. Some combinations may make you feel worse; others may make you feel better. If you're feeling worse, don't simply continue with the regimen or just give up — go back to your doctor and discuss the situation. While you're working the kinks out of your HT program, monitor your symptoms and any adverse reactions and write them down. Having some notes when you visit your doctor can help make the meeting more productive. You can accurately describe the symptoms and reactions to your doctor, and the two of you can come up with a treatment plan that works for you.

Remember that it may take your doctor time and you may have to try a couple of different formulas to find the correct therapy for you. Remember the lesson of the hospital gown — one size fits no one. If you're not comfortable with your doctor, find a medical advisor with whom you can work.

Quitting HT

If you're taking HT when you hit menopause, it may be a good time to re-evaluate your situation and consider the benefits you want to gain from hormone therapy. As you reconsider your decision, talk to your doctor. *Do not* simply stop taking HT. If you elect to quit taking HT, your doctor is the person in the best position to guide you.

Differences exist between the benefits and risks of long-term HT use and short-term HT use (see Tables 15-1 and 15-2 for a summary). The risks you're most worried about may not be a problem (or as big a problem) if you're taking HT for the short term — just long enough to get through the perimenopausal symptoms. With the recent study results in from the Women's Health Initiative, preventing cardiovascular disease no longer seems like a good reason to begin HT. To reduce heart disease and cardiovascular risks, start by improving your diet, getting more exercise, and quitting smoking. These methods are absolutely safe and proven to reduce your risk of cardiovascular problems (including heart attack and stroke).

After you make it through the hot flashes (with or without the use of HT) and you stop having periods, it's time to consider what you want to do about preventing health problems associated with sustained, low levels of estrogen. This is a good time to re-evaluate your regimen and consult with your healthcare advisor.

Finding Your Comfort Zone

This chapter takes a look at risk factors for various medical conditions that are associated with estrogen or the lack of it. But you can't make a decision about HT without considering your lifestyle and your personal preferences. Some women are frightened at the thought of taking another medication; others fear having a heart attack. Some women make a concerted effort to improve their health by committing to more exercise and a healthier diet; others are dedicated couch potatoes. Some women live in families who support new endeavors; others live in families who ridicule change. The following sections help you assess some of these touchy-feely personal values to see if you're likely to protect your health more successfully using diet, exercise, and non-HT alternatives or whether HT presents you with the best chances for success. Consider these factors as a piece of your HT decision-making puzzle.

Top ten (plus) signs that HT isn't for you

To get an HT program working for you, you have to communicate well with your doctor and share a sense of trust with him or her. If you aren't in that frame of mind, you may not have success with an HT program. And, if you're the type of woman who is wary of traditional medicine, pharmaceuticals, synthetic drugs, or all of the above, you may want try some of the alternatives to HT. You can always re-evaluate your condition and your comfort zone in the future.

Read the following statements and see if you agree with them. If you're in agreement with a lot of these statements, you may want to try HT alternatives including a healthy diet, exercise, herbal alternatives, and other preventative treatments.

1. I've had breast cancer

2. My mother, sister, or daughter has had breast cancer.

3. I have coronary heart disease.

4. I don't have or can live with my hot flashes, interrupted sleep, or other symptoms caused by hormonal changes.

5. I have a history of unexplained blood clots, deep-vein thrombosis, or blood clots in my lungs (*pulmonary embolism*).

6. I don't like taking medication and believe herbs can do a better job than drugs.

7. I typically eat a healthy diet that includes at least five servings of fruits and vegetables a day.

8. I exercise regularly, and I'm successful at maintaining my target weight.

9. I think physicians and pharmaceutical companies are just out to make money from women going through menopause.

10. I haven't gone to a doctor in years and don't plan on starting now.

11. My mother said she never had any problems going through menopause without hormones, and I don't think I will either.

12. I have very few risk factors for osteoporosis or cardiovascular disease.

Top ten signs that you're a good candidate for HT

No one wants to take medicine just to take it. Women who take HT during menopause are concerned about preventing disease or eliminating discomfort. To find a successful HT regimen, you must have confidence in your doctor and understand why you're making this decision because you may have to experiment for a while to find the right hormone regimen.

If you find yourself agreeing with some of these statements, you may want to consider HT.

1. I have a lot of osteoporosis in my family.

2. My mother or grandmother broke her hip.

3. I'm miserable with these hot flashes and mood swings, and my coworkers and family members are about to put me on a rocket bound for the moon.

4. I've been taking HT for a year now and haven't had any trouble.

5. I'm a junk-food junkie and could never survive on rabbit food like vegetables and fruit to stay fit.

6. My sex life is a huge problem because I'm not in the mood for it and intercourse is painful.

7. I don't have a huge number of risk factors for osteoporosis, but I've read the statistics, and I think that I'm at greater risk for that than breast cancer.

8. It seems like a lot of HT options exist, so I shouldn't have a problem sticking to a schedule.

9. I'm not big on herbal remedies to prevent or treat serious diseases.

10. I have a good rapport with my doctor, and I'd like to give HT a try to help prevent disease.

If you still have concerns or questions, talk to your physician. Don't simply stop a therapy you're presently taking. Your medical advisor may be able to help you interpret the information you read about a study. Don't base your decision about HT — or any medication, for that matter — on TV commercials or newspaper articles.

Figuring out just how bad it really is

This little quiz is designed to help you decide whether you're experiencing perimenopausal symptoms, and if so, whether they're interfering with your quality of life. The responses are ranked in order from least debilitating to most. The more debilitating, the greater the chance that these symptoms are interfering with your life. There are no cutoff points and no target scores — you be the judge.

How often do you experience hot flashes or night sweats?

✔ Never.

✔ Several times a week, but I can deal with it.

✔ Several times a day, and they interfere with my activities.

✔ So often that I'm going nuts.

How often do you experience interrupted sleep or insomnia?

✔ About the same as I have in the past.

✔ Once in a while, but I simply don't sleep as well as I used to.

✔ I wake up a couple times a night, and I have a hard time getting back to sleep.

✔ I feel like a zombie because I'm awake so much of the night.

Do you feel irritable, anxious, or apprehensive?

✔ No more than usual.

✔ I'm more irritable, anxious, or apprehensive than I used to be.

✔ I sometimes cry at the drop of a hat, and other times, I just want to be alone.

✔ I'm driving my family and coworkers nuts because I fly into a rage one minute and I'm fine the next.

Are you experiencing vaginal dryness, burning, or itching?

✔ No more than usual.

✔ Intercourse is uncomfortable at times.

✔ My partner and I have cut down on intercourse because it's painful, and I still feel itchy and uncomfortable.

✔ My vagina feels uncomfortable and itchy when doing everyday activities.

Do you experience any other perimenopausal problems? (Circle all that apply.)

✔ I experience perimenopausal-like symptoms prior to my period, but then, they go away.

✔ I've noticed my headaches are getting more frequent.

✔ My skin feels prickly, like bugs are crawling on me.

✔ I leak urine when I laugh, exercise, or sneeze.

✔ I seem to leak urine no matter what type of activity I'm doing.

✔ I have frequent memory lapses and have a hard time concentrating.

✔ My heartbeat flutters or pounds rapidly, sometimes when I'm just sitting or resting.

If you experience many of these symptoms but they appear at about the same time each month — prior to your period — and then go away for some length of time during each menstrual cycle, you probably have premenstrual syndrome rather than perimenopausal symptoms.

Chapter 16

Taking an Alternate Route: Non-Hormone Therapies

At least one-third of perimenopausal and menopausal women in the United States use some form of *nonconventional therapy* (medical therapies not commonly used or previously accepted in conventional Western medicine) to treat their symptoms.

If you're using (or considering using) nonconventional therapy, let your physician know about the products involved because natural supplements are still medicines — they can alter your physiology as much as medications from a pharmacy. (For example, some herbs used to treat menopausal symptoms interfere with anesthesia during a surgical procedure.) Treat these nonconventional approaches as seriously as you treat other medications.

The best way to approach nontraditional therapy is to use it in conjunction with traditional medicine — each approach has benefits and problems. We devote a number of chapters in this book to hormone therapy (HT) and traditional approaches to dealing with the symptoms of perimenopause and menopause, but in this chapter, we fill in the rest of the equation. We use this chapter to introduce you to nontraditional approaches — herbs, other plant-based therapies, mind-body therapies, biofeedback, and acupuncture. But first, we review the general opinions of medical professionals and groups concerning alternative treatments that focus on herbs and other plants.

If eliminating the annoying symptoms of perimenopause were all that it took to keep women healthy (and if the alternative therapies worked reliably and effectively on all women), alternative therapies would be the best bet because they generally have fewer complications and risks when compared to hormone therapies. But staying healthy during perimenopause and menopause requires the prevention of more serious health issues that begin when your body starts producing lower levels of estrogen.

Plowing through the Pros and Cons of Herbs

Interest in nonconventional therapy is growing. Some women enjoy taking a more holistic approach to their lives, menopause included, and others have made the choice to avoid at least some forms of conventional medicine and hormone therapy for various reasons. In this section, we detail why medical types are concerned about herbal therapies and how herbal therapies are becoming safer.

Complementary and *alternative medicines* are the names we use to refer to nonconventional therapies in this chapter. These names are just fancy ways to refer to a variety of practices and products that haven't always been considered part of conventional medicine.

These nonconventional therapies are called *complementary* if you use them in addition to conventional medicine and *alternative* if you use them in place of conventional medicine. For example, many women who take HT also use biofeedback to further reduce stress and anxiety. In this case, biofeedback is considered complementary treatment. (For more on biofeedback, see the "Tuning in to biofeedback" section later in this chapter.) An example of an alternative therapy is using black cohosh (an herb you can read about in the "Black cohosh" section later in this chapter) to relieve perimenopausal symptoms instead of using hormones.

Although we still use these terms, some therapies that were once considered nonconventional are sometimes incorporated into conventional medicine after years of research and success in treatment. Nonconventional courses of treatment have become so popular that the U.S. government (in the form of the National Institutes of Health; Internet: www.nih.gov) is now spending money on researching herbal and mind-body therapies like the ones we discuss in this chapter. Today, safely exploring these types of treatment is becoming easier and easier.

Taking conventional medicine's concerns into account

The biggest complaints voiced by conventional medicine concerning herb-based alternative treatments deal with the lack of scientific studies surrounding the plants. Some herbs have been studied in controlled experiments, but many have not, so researchers aren't sure whether they work any better than a sugar pill. Some therapies have been scrutinized more carefully than others, and if they work for you, that's great.

Any herb or plant therapy marketed and sold as a *medicine* in the United States must go through a U.S. Food and Drug Administration (FDA) approval process just like all other medicines (from antacids to cancer drugs). This approval process requires rigorous testing and trials. But few manufacturers of herbal therapies want to go through that process for an herb because plants can't be patented. If they spend the money to test the product and the product passes FDA muster, without a patent, competitors can copy their formula (harvest the herb and put it in a bottle). So, most manufacturers sell their products as *supplements.* Because supplements don't go through the FDA process, little proof or certification verifies that these therapies actually improve conditions as advertised and *cause no harm.*

The "cause no harm" part of the previous statement is very important. Herbs can be just as dangerous and toxic as drugs. They can interact with other medications you're currently taking. And they can produce toxic effects if taken in large quantities. Because most herbs aren't tested in recognized studies, warnings about side effects from taking an herb or too much of an herb are often sketchy, anecdotal, and not based on clinical trials. Chemicals that may be toxic are sometimes included within an herbal supplement (see the "Avoiding Problems with Plants" section later in this chapter for more info). When people ingest the herbs, they may also ingest toxic additives. The Web site of the National Center for Complementary and Alternative Medicine (www.nccam.nih.gov) has a special alert and advisory section to let you know the latest news concerning toxic effects of herbal treatments.

Conventional medicine's other complaint concerns testing for proper doses of the herbs. Many herbs are delivered to market without thorough tests of the effects of taking too large of a dose or taking the recommended dose for a long time.

When labels mention *recommended doses,* the definition of that term is often unclear. Who exactly is that dose recommended for — a person who weighs 150 pounds or a person who weighs 300 pounds? Should you take more of the supplement if your symptoms are more severe and less if they're less severe?

Is there an upper threshold at which the herb becomes toxic or a lower threshold at which the herb is ineffective? Do they interfere with drugs you're currently taking?

Also, consumers often have no means of measuring the exact quantity provided in a dose. Because the FDA doesn't have to approve supplements in the United States, manufacturers are under no requirement to label the amount of drug contained in the herbal supplement.

Growing safety into herbal therapy

Before picking up a bottle of herbs off the shelf in a health-food store or incorporating herbal therapies into your life, get assistance from a qualified herbalist. Qualified herbalists are likely to have experience in predicting herbal therapies that will work for you — a great alternative to playing the eeny-meeny-miney-mo game at the health-food store. An herbalist can help you find herbs that work well together and avoid combinations that have counterproductive or toxic effects.

To find an herbalist, consult one of the many herbalist organizations (take a look in Appendix B for more info). Most of these professional organizations have codes of ethics to which members must adhere and certification programs for their members. When looking for an herbalist, take all the investigative steps you would take if you were looking for a new doctor — talk to friends and interview the herbalist to find out about his or her training, practices, philosophy, and experience. An herbalist can help you put your shopping list together to make sure your therapy is as safe and effective as possible.

Research into the safety and effectiveness of herbs is much more advanced in Germany than it is in North America, and Germany has relatively strict guidelines for regulating herbal supplements. If possible, buy herbs that have been certified in Germany because herbal therapies that meet German standards are more reliable in terms of labeling the contents and the amount of active ingredients contained in each dose.

German health authorities use the guideline of *reasonable certainty,* which means that they consider the experiences of general practitioners — not just clinical trials — in evaluating a plant drug. *The Complete German Commission E Monographs: Therapeutic Guide to Herbal Medicines* (by Mark Blumenthal, published by Integrative Medicine Communications) is an English translation of the German "safe herb" list (the Commission E report). For more information on herbs, you can also check out *Herbal Remedies For Dummies* (Christopher Hobbs, Wiley Publishing, Inc.).

Relieving Your Symptoms with Plants

Herbal treatments for the mental, emotional, and physical symptoms associated with perimenopause and menopause abound. (A lot of these herbal treatments also relieve similar premenstrual-syndrome symptoms as well.) Herbalists use a number of botanical therapies that are mild, effective, and reliable. Some therapies have been tested in clinical trials; others have proven helpful through years of use.

Cataloging herbal therapies by symptom

If you're wondering what herbal therapy can do for you, here are some of the symptoms that perimenopausal and menopausal women look to herbs to relieve and the herbs that may be effective:

- **Depression and anxiety:** *Angelica sinensis, Eleutherococcus senticosus, Ginkgo biloba, Glycyrrhiza glabra, Hypericum perforatum, Leonorus cardiaca, Panax ginseng, Verbena hastate, Withania somnifera*

- **Heart palpitations:** *Cimicifuga racemosa, Crataegus oxyacanth, Leonorus cardiaca*

- **Heavy bleeding:** *Achillea millefolium, Alchemilla vulgaris, Capsella bursa-pastoris, Myrica cerifera*

- **Hot flashes and night sweats:** *Actea racemosa, Leonorus cardiaca, Panax ginseng, Salvia officinalis*

- **Insomnia:** *Eleutherococcus senticosus, Glycyrrhiza glabra, Lavendula officinalis, Leonorus cardiac, Passiflora incarnata, Piper methysticum, Scutellaria lateriflora, Valeriana officinalis, Withania somnifera,*

- **Memory problems:** *Bacopa moniera, Paeonia lactiflora, Panax ginseng, Gingko biloba, Rosmarinus officinalis*

- **Vaginal dryness:** *Actaea racemosa, Calendula officinalis, Glycyrrhiza glabra, Panax quinquefolium, Trifolium pratense*

We don't claim to be herbalists, but we do know that women in Europe and Asia have used some herbs for years to treat the symptoms of perimenopause and menopause. However, we give no advice as to dosage for a couple of reasons:

1. The quantity of active ingredients varies from brand to brand.

2. You should always seek help from a qualified herbalist before taking herbs.

Herbs are natural, but natural doesn't mean that they're without side effects.

Getting the scoop on individual herbs

Many of the herbs used to treat perimenopausal and menopausal symptoms are phytoestrogens (*phyto* means plant, and you know what estrogen is). *Phytoestrogens* are plant estrogens — natural sources of estrogen that act as weak estrogens and seem to produce estrogen effects in menopausal women. In other words, they reduce perimenopausal and menopausal symptoms.

If you take phytoestrogens without a progestin, you're at a higher risk for endometrial cancer. Phytoestrogens are natural, but they still are mild forms of estrogen and cause your uterine lining to continue to thicken. If you use these herbs, simply mention it to your doctor. He or she can monitor your bleeding and perform tests or recommend therapy as needed. (For more information on unopposed estrogen therapy, see Chapter 10.)

Please tell your doctor if you're taking any of these herbs. Some of them interfere the effectiveness of other medicines. They're considered medicines when your doctor asks you, "What medicines are you taking?"

Ashwagandha (Withania somnifera)

Much like ginseng, eleuthero, and licorice, ashwagandha is said to reduce stress and depression and aid sleep with long-term use.

Black cohosh (Actaea racemosa syn, Cimicifuga racemosa)

Women have used black cohosh for hundreds, maybe thousands, of years. (Early Native Americans used black cohosh, and other folk medicines made use of it.) Today it's one of the more commonly used phytoestrogens in the battle against perimenopausal symptoms because it relieves hot flashes, vaginal atrophy, tension, elevated blood pressure, restless sleep, and stress.

Again, black cohosh is a phytoestrogen, so talk to your doctor before using it if you have breast cancer or if you plan on using it for more than three or four months.

If you're going to give black cohosh a try, you can find it sold under the brand name Remifemin. Remifemin is the extract approved in Germany to treat menopause, and it seems to have fewer side effects than other formulas. The German recommendation is to use it for six months or less (to avoid thickening of your endometrium).

Dong Quai (Angelica sinensis)

Also known as *tang gui,* this herb has been used for hundreds of years in traditional Chinese medicine to "strengthen the blood." Dong quai is the natural form of Coumadin (generic name: warfarin), a "blood-thinner" drug doctors often prescribe for women who have *arrhythmia* (irregular heart beat) because it dilates the blood vessels and decreases clotting to improve blood flow to your heart. It also seems to eliminate hot flashes.

Possible drawbacks? Dong quai reduces blood clotting, so if you're having surgery be sure to let your doctor know beforehand that you've been using this herb. You should stop using it two weeks before surgery. Also, don't use dong quai if you've had unexplained vaginal bleeding. Try to avoid aspirin and other drugs that serve to thin your blood while using this herb.

Ginkgo (Gingko biloba)

Here's one that's been in the news quite a bit. This herb is said to improve your memory and feeling of well-being, and one study of 200 women showed that it increased sexual desire.

But don't use it with abandon. Ginkgo reduces blood clotting (it thins your blood), so be sure to let your doctor know that you're using this herb. If you're scheduled to undergo an operation, quit taking ginko at least two weeks before surgery. And don't take it if you're taking other blood thinners such as the drug Coumadin (or the herb dong quai).

Ginseng (Panax ginseng, Panax quinqafolium)

People all over the world consume ginseng to increase vitality, improve memory, relieve anxiety, and kick start low libido. Historically, menopausal women have used ginseng to relieve depression, fatigue, memory lapses, and low libido. It doesn't seem to raise your estrogen levels or cause your endometrium to thicken as some of the phytoestrogens tend to do.

You have to be careful about using ginseng if you're taking other types of medication for depression or anxiety. It's been known to cause mania when combined with certain antidepressant medications.

Kava (Piper methysticum)

Herbalists use kava to reduce anxiety and chronic pain and to promote sleep and relaxation. However, even herbalists recognize a need for further tests to determine if this herb is potentially toxic to the liver.

This herb may be harmful to your liver. Talk to your doctor if you choose to take it.

Motherwort (Leonorus cardiaca)

The Chinese have used motherwort for a long time. Western herbalists make use of it to treat menopausal anxiety, insomnia, heart palpitations, and vaginal atrophy.

Peony (Paeonia lactiflora)

Peony helps dilate the blood vessels so that blood flows more smoothly through your cardiovascular system. Some folks claim that it also improves your mental focus and reduces mental lapses.

Red clover (Trifolium pratense)

Menopausal women often find that this herb, historically used to treat skin and breathing problems, relieves vaginal dryness and lowers their LDL ("bad" cholesterol) levels while increasing their HDL (the good stuff) levels. Red clover contains *isoflavones* (the chemicals that make phytoestrogens work like estrogen), so it acts as a mild estrogen.

As with all phytoestrogens, don't use red clover if you have breast cancer.

Sage (Salvia officinalis)

Sage is said to relieve hot flashes, but the claim hasn't been widely researched.

Saint John's wort (Hypericum perforatum)

The popularity of Saint John's wort for treating depression has grown tremendously in recent years, but people have used this herb since the Middle Ages. During perimenopause and menopause, women use it to treat mild depression. Although a lot of published reports show that Saint John's wort does work, how it works is a question that we don't have an answer for.

This herb can cause sensitivity to light. It also interferes with a variety of other medications, so as with any herb, tell your doctor that you're taking it.

Soy

Soy is a plant estrogen (phytoestrogen), so it has the same pluses and problems as other phytoestrogens. It's reported to relieve hot flashes, interrupted sleep, anxiety, and other perimenopausal symptoms. However, too much soy has the same effect as unopposed estrogen (unfettered thickening of the uterine lining).

Although many advertisements for soy products point to the health of women in Japan and China as evidence that they work, women in these cultures start eating soy early in life, and they eat mostly fermented-soy products, such as *miso* (soybean paste) and *tempeh* (a cheese-like soybean food), rather than soy-protein drinks and milk. But studies have shown that soy can clean up your blood by reducing your total cholesterol, LDL cholesterol (the bad cholesterol), triglycerides, and blood pressure while raising your HDL (the good cholesterol) levels.

Vitex (Vitex agnus castus)

Vitex, or *chaste tree,* acts like progesterone by helping to reduce peri-menopausal stress and depression (Some women have found that it does just the opposite, but reports of vitex causing stress and depression are rare.) Because it acts like progesterone, vitex may help stabilize the uterine lining. Herbalists say that it's safe for long-term use.

Avoiding Problems with Plants

As we state throughout this chapter, just because herbs are natural doesn't mean they're safe. People get into trouble with herbs because they don't real-ize that herbs are drugs that produce both positive and negative effects. Some people with certain medical conditions are more susceptible to side effects associated with some herbs. For example, women with cardiovascular disease should be careful with herbs because the containers don't necessarily carry any warning. Here are some other things to look out for when using herbs:

✔ Some herbs can damage your liver causing chronic hepatitis or acute liver injury. These herbs include chaparral, comfrey, coltsfoot, germander, Gordolobo yerba tea, mate tea, pennyroyal oil (also known as squaw mint), and many others.

✔ Therapies that contain the active ingredient *mefanamic acid* can cause liver and kidney damage (and sometimes your kidneys quit functioning altogether, which spells trouble).

✔ Any herb or supplement that includes *ephedra* or caffeine is dangerous for women with high blood pressure or cardiovascular disease. (The Chinese herb *mahuang* is the same thing as ephedra.) Unfortunately caffeine is often added to tonics and supplements without being listed on the label.

If you feel heart palpitations or anxiety with any herbal therapy, stop using it immediately.

Getting Touchy about Acupuncture

Acupuncture is a form of Chinese medicine in which an acupuncturist inserts needles into specific points along critical energy paths in your body. For the doubters out there, acupuncture isn't all that far out. Asian doctors have successfully performed surgeries using acupuncture as the anesthesia.

Acupuncture stimulates your body's ability to resist or overcome menopausal symptoms by correcting energy imbalances. Acupuncture also prompts your body to produce chemicals that decrease or eliminate pain and discomfort.

Acupuncturists place fine needles into your body, which affect your *chi* — your life-force energy that travels through pathways in your body that are called *meridians*. Acupuncturists have mapped out the meridians and specific points along the meridians in the human body, so they know where to place the needle given your specific symptoms. You tell the acupuncturist your symptoms — heavy bleeding, headaches, and hot flashes, for example — and he or she knows exactly how to place the needles to relieve your discomfort.

Acupuncture is recognized as a legitimate form of complementary or alternative medicine, and many insurance plans cover this type of therapy. If you're interested in trying this therapy, find a qualified specialist. Many states regulate and license acupuncturists, so you can probably get names of licensed acupuncturists from your state department of health.

Soothing Symptoms with Relaxation Therapies

Stress can be great if it motivates you to do your best — like in a race. But, if you're continually stressed out, stress can actually do physical damage to your mind and body. It can lead to excessive eating, sleeplessness (not only in Seattle), anxiety, depression, and irritability. (Do any of these symptoms sound familiar — as in perimenopausal and menopausal symptoms?) Continued stress can also affect your immune system, making you more susceptible to cancer, hypertension, heart problems, and headaches — the medical concerns women worry about after menopause.

Take a look at some of these nonmedical therapies that can help you relax and reduce the stress in your life. With stress, like Brylcreem, "A little dab will do you."

Tuning in to biofeedback

Biofeedback relies on the interconnectedness of the mind and body. Back in the 1600s, to appease the Christian church, medical pioneers drew an artificial line between the body and the spirit and told religious leaders that medicine would concern itself only with the physical body. Centuries later, Western medicine is trying to reunite the mind and body in their proper interconnected context in order to make our approaches to healing more comprehensive.

Biofeedback has been around since the 1960s, but it uses some of the mind-body lessons taught by ancient martial arts. The biggest difference between biofeedback and the martial arts is technology. Biofeedback uses monitoring instruments to provide you with physiological information (feedback) — information you otherwise wouldn't be aware of. By watching the monitoring device, and through trial and error, you learn to adjust your thinking and mental attitudes to control bodily processes that folks used to think were involuntary. Using biofeedback, some people learn to control blood pressure, temperature, gastrointestinal functioning, and brainwave activity.

Some of the menopause-related conditions you can treat with biofeedback are

- Hypertension
- Migraine headaches
- Sleep difficulties
- Stress
- Urinary incontinence

Getting your yoga groove on

Now here's a great way to kill two birds with one stone. Yoga can help you improve your flexibility (something that starts decreasing after you've been on this planet for about 35 years) and relieve stress. Staying flexible is an important part of balance; so being flexible reduces your chance of falling and breaking a bone. Reducing stress improves your immunity by helping you avoid disease and also improve your mental outlook.

Yoga is also a great way to keep your bones strong and improve your muscle tone. Yoga combines breathing, meditation, and stretching techniques to help strengthen bones and muscles and improve posture, breathing, oxygen flow, relaxation, and overall health and vitality. Take a class or grab a book — many different forms of yoga are out there, and it's great for women of all ages.

Slip Sliding Away with Topical Treatments

Many perimenopausal and menopausal women experience *vaginal atrophy* (drying and thinning of the vagina). You can treat this condition in several ways without using hormone therapy.

You can buy lubricants without a prescription in the grocery store that will help relieve the day-to-day discomfort of vaginal dryness. Replens is one of the more popular brands of lubricants and has shown to be as effective as vaginal estrogen cream in relieving vaginal dryness in tests. Replens comes in a tube with an applicator. You simply fill the applicator, insert the tube into your vagina, and press the applicator. You do this once a week.

In addition to over-the-counter lubricants, some of the herbs we discuss in this chapter also relieve vaginal dryness. (Check out the "Cataloging herbal therapies by symptom" section earlier in this chapter.)

If vaginal atrophy is causing painful intercourse, we have a prescription-free solution for you. A number of lubricants are designed to help you get slippery. In fact, you may find that sex is more fun when you "butter up" than it was before. K-Y Jelly has been around for years. Hospitals and doctors' offices use it for lubricating thermometers when taking temperatures rectally and for many other purposes. It also works well as a lubricant before intercourse. Astroglide is another terrific product that can make you more slippery. You can rub all of these products on your vagina prior to intercourse.

Chapter 17

Treating Conditions without Hormone Therapy

. . . .

In This Chapter

▶ Beefing up your bones without estrogen

▶ Heading towards a healthy heart without hormones

. . . .

*P*rolonged periods of low estrogen levels can promote bone deterioration and cardiovascular conditions. Although many women choose to use hormone therapy (HT) to prevent these issues, other medications and therapies that directly treat these issues are available. The treatments we discuss in this chapter are targeted to specific conditions or diseases. Hormone therapy tries to treat these conditions indirectly by adjusting hormone levels. Whether or not you use hormones, you can use the treatments we cover in this chapter. Some of the treatments are medications; others are lifestyle choices.

Battling Bone Loss and Osteoporosis with Medication

One of the best ways to avoid *osteoporosis* (brittle bone disease) is to start out with strong, healthy bones. You can accomplish this feat by getting plenty of calcium and vitamins D and K in your diet during childhood, adolescence, and early adulthood. (For the complete lowdown on caring for your bones, check out Chapter 4.) Of course, hindsight is 20/20, and it may be too late at this point in your life to start developing healthy bone mass. (But it may not be too late for the young women in your life, so spread the word.) Fear not: In the following sections, we outline some other ways to improve the health of your bones during menopause without using HT.

A number of drugs can help preserve bone density. The drugs we mention in this chapter, taken in combination with a healthy diet and exercise programs, can slow the rate of bone loss and, in many cases, actually increase bone density over time.

Talking bisphosphonates

A group of drugs called *bisphosphonates* are the most effective medications for halting and reversing bone loss in menopausal women. These drugs work by slowing down the destruction part (*resorption*) of the bone-maintenance process. The following list contains some examples of bisphosphonates. Unless otherwise noted, we list the drugs by their brand names followed by the generic names in parentheses.

✔ **Fosamax (alendronate):** This medication is one of the most commonly used bisphosphonates. Approved by the Food and Drug Administration for use in the United States in 1995, Fosamax prevents bone material from breaking down, and it actually builds stronger bones. When you include this medication as part of a healthy lifestyle (enough calcium and regular exercise), you can cut your risk of fracture in half. Like all medications, this drug comes with some rules. You have to

- **Take it first thing in the morning on a completely empty stomach.** You may have to adjust your morning schedule if you like to hop out of bed and into the coffee pot.

- **Take it with a full glass of water.** Don't substitute coffee, juice, cola, or anything else. Use plain water.

- **Remain upright after taking it.** Sorry, but you can't go back to bed. If you don't remain upright after you take it, Fosamax can cause a reflux type of reaction in which you have a burning sensation in your esophagus.

- **Wait for an hour after taking it before you eat breakfast.** Actually the longer you wait to eat or drink anything, the better your body absorbs the medication. Waiting two hours before eating is even better than waiting just one. If you wait two hours, your body absorbs nearly 70 percent of the drug, but if you only wait 30 minutes, the number drops to about 46 percent. If you eat when you take Fosamax, you won't absorb enough of the medication to help your bones.

This drug comes in once-a-day and once-a-week pill form. Fosamax presents very few side effects when you take it correctly. Women who are taking hormone therapy can use this drug to get even more protection from fracture.

✔ **Actonel (risedronate):** This bisphosphonate received approval for use in the United States for preventing and treating osteoporosis in early 2000. Actonel is supposed to have fewer gastrointestinal side effects than Fosamax presents, and it has a slightly better track record in reducing the risk of fracture (65 percent reduction in the risk of fracture for Actonel versus 47 percent for Fosamax). Actonel comes in once-a-day or once-a-week pill form. You can take this medication even if you take hormone therapy.

Introducing calcitonin

Miacalcin (calcitonin) is a nasal spray that uses a different technique to slow down bone loss than the bisphosphonates use. Calcitonin is actually a hormone that occurs naturally in your body. It helps regulate your calcium levels by slowing the rate of bone deterioration. It also relieves bone pain caused by osteoporosis.

The rules with this stuff are a bit simpler but still pretty specific. You use one squirt in one nostril per day, alternating nostrils on a daily basis. (Is this a cruel joke or what? Don't the Miacalcin bigwigs know that menopausal women often experience memory lapses?) Calcitonin isn't quite as effective at preventing bone loss as the bisphosphonates, but it may reduce the pain of existing spinal fractures.

Considering fluoride

Fluoride stimulates bone building, but the bone it builds seems to be brittle. All the bisphosphonates treat osteoporosis by slowing down the natural bone destruction process, but fluoride works on the other side of the bone-maintenance equation by aiding the formation of new bone.

Although fluoride increases bone density, it doesn't reduce fractures. After reading that statement, you may be thinking, "What good is thick bone if it's not strong?" Good question. That's why fluoride isn't normally used to treat osteoporosis. Some new research is being conducted using slow-release fluoride along with calcium supplements to see if stronger bone can be built. Stay tuned for more.

Controlling Cardiovascular Disease

Cardiovascular disease includes conditions that affect the blood, blood vessels, or heart (otherwise known as the cardiovascular system). (For more information on how this system works see Chapter 5.) Controlling cardiovascular disease is the big one. Reducing the risks of cardiovascular disease was thought to be one of the biggest benefits of HT, but the results of the Women's Health Initiative study have called all that into question. (See Chapter 11 for the lowdown on this issue.)

The risks of cardiovascular disease are high for women after menopause — nearly one out of every two women in the United States will die of some type of cardiovascular disease. Given the high incidence of cardiovascular disease in women over 50 and the controversy over whether hormone therapy increases or decreases your risk, you *really* need to put some thought into how to keep your blood, blood vessels, and heart healthy for the next 40 or 50 years. In the following sections, we provide you with some strategies.

Reducing your risk of heart attack with drugs

Half of all heart attacks occur in people with normal cholesterol levels, so a healthy cholesterol profile doesn't mean you're out of the woods. Of course, the other side of that story is that half of all heart attacks occur in people with lousy cholesterol profiles. So try to maintain a healthy diet and exercise program and take your cholesterol medication if your doctor recommends it.

Arteriosclerosis (clogged arteries) isn't the only problem that triggers a heart attack. Many other conditions can lead to a heart attack as well:

- ✔ Angina (blood vessel spasms)
- ✔ Arrhythmia (irregular heart beat)
- ✔ Blood clots
- ✔ High blood pressure

To reduce your risk of heart attack, be sure to maintain a healthy diet, exercise regularly, and take the medication your doctor prescribes to treat high cholesterol and any of these cardiovascular conditions. The following are other medications used to control or prevent heart attack:

- ✔ **ACE inhibitors:** Docs often use ACE inhibitors on people who have recently had a heart attack and who have heart failure or decreased function of the left ventricle. If used within 24 hours of the start of heart-attack symptoms, ACE inhibitors can keep you from dying of the heart attack and prevent heart failure stemming from the heart attack. The "ACE" part stands for *angiotensin-converting enzyme* — we threw that in here just in case you're a big fan of medical terms.

✔ **Aspirin:** Recently people have started paying a whole lot of renewed attention to this trusted pain reliever. The buzz surrounds aspirin's ability to lower the risk of heart attack when taken every day. Aspirin performs this function by keeping your *platelets* (special blood cells responsible for clotting) from sticking together too much and forming blood clots unnecessarily. Aspirin is what's known as an *anticoagulant* (it keeps your blood from coagulating, or clotting). If your body starts forming clots too readily, the clots can clog your blood vessels and lead to heart attack or stroke. If you have angina, your doctor may recommend aspirin to avoid a heart attack. Or if you've already had a heart attack, your doctor may recommend that you take aspirin daily to avoid another attack.

Even though aspirin is an over-the-counter medication, it can have dangerous side effects. Read the warning label on the bottle and discuss possible side effects with your doctor. And even though preventing blood clots with aspirin can help you avoid a heart attack, blood clotting is an important bodily function that stops you from bleeding if you cut yourself or have surgery. Be sure to tell your doctor that you're taking aspirin regularly if you're facing surgery.

✔ **Coumadin:** You may see this drug referred to by its generic name, warfarin. Coumadin is another drug doctors use to prevent blood from clotting. But unlike aspirin, it's a prescription drug. Coumadin is more effective than aspirin in preventing blood clots, so you must use caution and have your blood monitored regularly when taking it. Women who have angina or who have irregular heartbeats often take this medication to help move blood more fluidly through the vessels.

✔ **Thrombolytics:** Doctors give a member of this class of drugs to patients having a heart attack because of a blood clot. Thrombolytics can dissolve a clot and restore blood flow to the heart. These drugs must be administered within six hours of the heart attack (before heart tissue begins to die from lack of oxygen) to be effective.

✔ **Vasodilators:** These drugs help blood vessels relax and dilate (widen) so that your heart doesn't have to work as hard to get oxygen-rich blood into the heart muscle. *Nitroglycerin* is a common vasodilator given to women who suffer from angina. Take these drugs as directed by your doctor.

Treating high blood pressure with drugs

A variety of drugs are available today that treat hypertension (high blood pressure). They fall into two main categories:

- **Beta-blockers:** A number of different types of beta-blockers are sold under a variety of brand names. These drugs reduce your heart rate and blood pressure. Sometimes doctors also prescribe them to treat angina.

- **Calcium channel blockers:** These drugs reduce your heart's oxygen requirements, increase the blood supply to your heart, and lower blood pressure. They can prevent coronary artery spasms if you have angina.

Keeping your blood lean and mean with drugs

Blood that's high in LDL cholesterol (the bad stuff) and triglycerides encourages the fat and cholesterol to build up in the lining of your blood vessels, which leads to *arteriosclerosis* (hardening of the arteries) and can eventually cause a heart attack (see Chapter 5 for the entire story).

But some medications can lower bad cholesterol (LDL) and triglyceride levels and raise good cholesterol (HDL) levels. These medications are called *antilipemic drugs* because they help moderate your lipid levels (cholesterol and triglycerides). Here's what the National Cholesterol Education Program recommends to keep your cholesterol levels in check and to keep your cardiovascular system healthy:

- Get your blood cholesterol levels checked every year (total cholesterol, LDL, HDL, and triglycerides). For more information on blood cholesterol tests see Chapter 5.

- Visit your doctor regularly to assess your risk of cardiovascular problems.

- Read the labels on your foods and choose foods that are low in saturated fat and cholesterol.

- Keep your weight in check (turn to Chapter 18 for more on weighty issues).

- Exercise regularly (see Chapter 19 for recommendations).

- Don't smoke and avoid second-hand smoke.

If changes in your diet, activity level, and lifestyle don't improve your cholesterol levels, your doctor may recommend medication to improve your cholesterol profile. Several types of drugs are available to lower cholesterol:

- **Bile acid sequestrants:** These drugs lower LDL levels and can be used alone or in combination with statin drugs.

- **Fibric acids:** Fibric acids lower LDL levels a bit but are usually used to treat high-triglyceride and low-HDL levels.

- **Nicotinic acid:** This babies lower LDL and triglyceride levels and raise HDL levels.

- **Statins:** These drugs are very effective in lowering LDL levels.

Your doctor is the only person who can determine if cholesterol-lowering drugs are right for you and which type of drugs can meet your needs.

Living a hearty lifestyle

Here's a simple fact: Study after study has shown that smoking absolutely increases your risk of cardiovascular problems because it promotes the buildup of fat and cholesterol in your arteries and increases the formation of blood clots that can cause heart attacks. Eliminating smoking is a good way to lower your risk of cardiovascular disease. Your risk begins to drop immediately after you quit. By your tenth anniversary of beginning a smoke-free life, your risk of cardiovascular disease is similar to that of a woman who never smoked.

Smoking isn't the only enemy of cardiovascular health. Weight matters. Gaining more than 12 to 18 pounds after age 18 increases your risk of coronary heart disease, and your risk becomes greater as you gain more weight. If you've gained 40 or more pounds since your 18th birthday, you've doubled your risk of heart disease. If you want to look at the connection in a more positive light, you'll be glad to know that your cholesterol drops 25 points with every 10 pounds you lose.

A life full of anger, anxiety, depression, and isolation also increases your risk of cardiovascular disease. If one or more of these emotional conditions rule your life, it's not healthy, especially for your cardiovascular system. Having a network of friends or relatives who can offer you emotional support can lower your risk of cardiovascular disease. Try meditation or physical activity to reduce anger, depression, and anxiety. You may want to share your symptoms with a healthcare provider in order to begin treating them.

Picking a heart-healthy diet

The National Cancer Institute recommends eating at least five fruits and vegetables each day to reduce your risk of heart disease (and cancer). "Get five to survive, but nine is divine" is a slogan used by the Cooper Institute, one of the most prestigious preventative-health institutions in the world. The institute is talking about the number of servings of fruits and vegetables you should consume *each day.* That means you need to spend less time in front of the dairy case and more time in the produce section at the grocery store. Five to nine servings of fruits and vegetables sounds like a lot, but meeting this goal is actually pretty easy. Check out Chapter 18 for dietary tips.

Part IV
Lifestyle Issues for Menopause and Beyond

The 5th Wave   By Rich Tennant

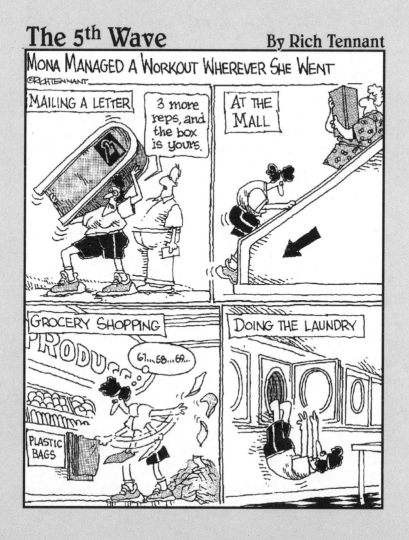

In this part . . .

Your body is changing. That's a fact. Your body is less forgiving about things like the pint of ice cream you just couldn't resist. That's a fact too. With all the changes going on, now is a perfect time to subscribe (or renew your subscription) to healthy habits like balancing your diet, getting a bit of physical activity, and breaking those bad-health habits. A few slight modifications in your daily routine can ensure that your body is living up to its potential. In this part, we offer practical advice that makes getting or staying fit before and after the change relatively easy. (And dare we say fun?)

Chapter 18

Eating for The Change

· ·

In This Chapter

▶ Brushing up on good eating habits

▶ Using nutrition to alleviate health problems

▶ Reaching and maintaining a healthy weight

· ·

*Y*ou've probably noticed that your body is less forgiving these days. In your twenties, you could order that extra glass of wine without paying for it in spades the next day. Back then, over-exercising meant sore muscles the next morning; now it takes two days of ibuprofen, hot showers, and a massage to feel better. And an injury can set you back twice as long now as it did when you were a twentysomething.

Menopause is your natural reminder that your body is aging and entering the prime time of some nasty health issues. Lower estrogen levels increase your risk of medical problems such as osteoporosis, cardiovascular disease, and more. A healthy diet and lifestyle can lower your risk for many of these medical issues, give you more energy, and improve your quality of life. It can also reduce some of the annoying symptoms of menopause, such as hot flashes.

Menopause gets your attention, up front and personal, with less than subtle physical reminders like hot flashes, weight shifting to your middle, heart palpitations, and the like. You can't help but take notice that your body is changing; and if you're ever going to get in shape, now's the time. Indeed, it's time to begin your preventive health care program so that you can continue to live an active and healthy life.

You also need to pay attention to your eating habits because taking off weight can be harder now than it used to be. With middle age, your metabolism starts to slow down. If you also decrease your physical activity, which some women do when they reach middle age, you'll find yourself gradually gaining weight. Lower estrogen levels also trigger redistribution of fat around your waist. That curvy pear shape turns into more of an apple shape as fat migrates to your middle.

In this chapter, we don't recommend any quick fixes. To stay healthy, you have to develop healthy *habits*. Habits are built on small changes that you can live with — without feeling as though you're making tremendous sacrifices. If you adopt healthier eating habits, you can avoid dieting and feel better. We don't have a miracle program; we just give you some great ways to eat healthier so you can get to a healthy weight, maintain it, and help reduce your risk of many diseases that strike menopausal women.

Eating to Promote Good Health

"You are what you eat" may sound trite, but it's true. Scientific evidence demonstrates that the foods you ingest affect your health, but you probably have real-life experiences that prove this point. During the major transformation that is menopause, you want maximum energy and protection from disease. A proper diet can help ensure success on both fronts.

How do you promote good health through your diet? By adopting or maintaining healthy eating habits. Many studies link healthy eating habits to good health. *Healthy eating habits* means eating a balanced diet of foods that keeps your body well nourished and able to fend off disease and environmental toxins.

Studies show that people who eat at least five helpings of fruit and vegetables each day cut their risk of stroke by nearly a third (and they also lessen their risk of cancer and heart disease). Another study found that the single most important factor in keeping the immune system healthy is a balanced diet.

Eating right helps your body fight off illness and protects your blood vessels, your bones, and your heart and other organs from chronic disease. Dieticians recommend that you eat five to ten servings of fruits and vegetables each day. Why? The antioxidants, phytochemicals, and fiber in fruits and vegetables build immunities, lower your blood pressure, and reduce your risk of heart disease, stroke, and many types of cancer.

Eating healthy is easier than you think. You don't have to walk around with a calorie-counting book. You don't have to eliminate all your favorite foods. You don't have to eliminate snacks. And you don't have to live solely on grapefruit juice and tofu. All you have to do is eat the right proportion of carbohydrates, protein, and fats and consume no more than 1,500 to 1,800 calories each day.

Here's a quick example of a simple fruit-and-veggie meal plan that provides five of these great foods in one day:

- ✔ **Breakfast:** A piece of fruit (like a banana or an orange)
- ✔ **Lunch:** A salad or fruit with your meal
- ✔ **Snack:** Another piece of fruit sometime during the day (like an apple)
- ✔ **Dinner:** A vegetable and a salad or two vegetables

Sneaking in the vegetables

We know that some folks aren't crazy about vegetables. If you're one of them, try these easy and painless tips for fitting more vegetables into your diet:

✔ **Add vegetables to sandwiches.** Try some lettuce, cucumbers, tomatoes, bell peppers, or sprouts. Remember that you only need ½ cup of veggies to count them as a serving.

✔ **Add chopped carrots, bell peppers, zucchini, or yellow squash to meatloaf.** These veggies make tasty additions, and vegetable-phobic folks barely notice them.

✔ **Add vegetables to your whole grain pasta.** Sauté garlic, onions, and chopped carrots or zucchini in a pan sprayed with vegetable

oil. When the pasta is tender, dump it in with the sautéed vegetables.

✔ **Combine a variety of colorful vegetables together.** You can stir-fry (spray vegetable oil on the pan instead of pouring it from the bottle to lower the amount of oil you use), roast (spray with vegetable oil and broil in the oven for 10 minutes), or grill the vegetables outside (forget the vegetable oil altogether) and then arrange them in colorful layers to make them visually appealing.

✔ **Add chopped vegetables to brown rice.** Peas, corn, broccoli, tomatoes, and bell peppers work well, but you can use any of your favorite vegetables.

See how easy that is? And besides, most people can find quite a few fruits and vegetables that they like to eat, so turning your diet in a healthier direction can be fun and enjoyable.

Trendy diets come and go — and then come back again with a new name. Forget about them. You don't need to follow the advice of some late-night, slick-talking, infomercial guru to eat healthy and achieve or maintain a healthy weight. A well-balanced diet will keep you full, and proper portion sizes along with exercise and planning will keep you at your preferred weight.

We list several great resources for those of you interested in eating healthier and losing weight or keeping it off in Appendix B.

Getting the right mix of nutrients

People eat for a lot of reasons other than to satisfy hunger. In fact, sometimes people eat even when they're not hungry (we're guilty and bet you are too, sometimes). You may eat for emotional reasons: out of boredom, because you're tired, angry, sad, happy — you name it. Sometimes certain environments trigger eating — you nibble as you clear the table, talk on the phone, or watch TV.

If you want to stay healthy and stick to a healthy weight, you need to eat with a purpose! Think of food like fuel. What do you need to keep your body fueled during the day? (The "fuel" is your blood sugar, which gives you the energy to build muscle, repair cells, and fight illness.) You need to feed your body the right mixture of proteins, complex carbohydrates, and fats to keep your well-tuned machine purring. Table 18-1 shows the breakdown for a healthy, balanced diet.

Table 18-1	Balancing the Scales of a Healthy Diet
Nutrient	*Percent of Daily Calories*
Protein	10–20
Complex carbohydrates	50–70
Fats	15–30

Based on American Heart Association dietary guidelines.

Proteins, carbohydrates, and fats work as a team to keep your energy level high and your body in good repair. Simple carbohydrates (like sugar) give you quick energy, but it only lasts a few minutes. Complex carbohydrates (like whole grains, fruits, and vegetables) fuel your body for one to three hours. Proteins provide energy over the course of four or five hours, and fats fuel your body for most of the day (five to six hours). Getting the right combination of foods throughout the day will give you energy and keep you from having sudden cravings or feeling tired, anxious, or sleepy.

Phytochemicals, plant nutrients that are still being researched, may protect against heart disease and cancer and build your immune system. They're found in red grapefruit, tomato, watermelon, lemons, and limes.

At any given meal, you don't want to include too much sugar (the energy you get only lasts 15 to 20 minutes, and you quickly become tired and hungry) or too much fat (provides lots of calories, but not enough short-term energy). If you get the right combination of protein, carbohydrates, and fats you'll feel fully charged for three to five hours.

The best way to approach this nutritional trio is to eat some foods belonging to each category during each meal, but if you can't manage that, make sure you achieve the proper proportion by the end of the day.

In addition to eating right, you need to drink plenty of fluids. Most dieticians recommend that you drink at least eight glasses of fluids a day, with at least four of those glasses being water. If you're increasing the fiber in your diet, you may want to drink a couple more glasses of water each day to help the flushing process. Coffee, tea, sugar-free hot chocolate, and sugar-free soft drinks help you keep your fluids up without tacking on too many extra calories.

If you blow it one day, don't stress out. If you find yourself regularly struggling to eat the right amounts of the right foods, try sitting down and planning out your meals for a few days at a time. Paying attention to what you eat helps you control your eating and weight.

Fine-tuning your carb intake (Carbohydrate, not carburetor)

The bulk of your diet should consist of complex carbohydrates, which works out well because fruits and vegetables — the food group you're supposed to eat five servings of each day — generally contain complex carbohydrates.

Simple carbohydrates

The quickest way to raise your blood sugar is to eat sugar (soft drinks, candy, jam). It takes very little effort for your body to take sugar and put it into your bloodstream.

These simple sugars give you a quick burst of energy, but your blood sugar drops just as quickly after about 15 minutes. Even athletes find that the quick rush of sugar doesn't do much to enhance their performance, so avoid these.

Complex carbohydrates

Think of complex carbohydrates as "plant foods" because they include fruits and vegetables as well as whole grains. They are digested more slowly than simple carbohydrates so they provide fuel over a longer period of time — one to three hours.

Choose fresh fruits and vegetables over the canned or processed variety because the fresh versions contain more nutrients and fiber and less sugar and salt. Choose whole-grain products (flours, breads, cereals, and so on) over refined or processed grains because a lot of the vitamins, minerals, and fiber are in the outer layer (the hull) of the grain, which is removed during processing.

Fiber is a type of complex carbohydrate and is sometimes called *roughage*. Fiber is simply plant material that doesn't break down in the human digestive system.

- **Soluble fiber** dissolves in water and is found in a variety of berries and other fruits as well as oats, legumes, and potatoes. Because they pass more slowly through your digestive system, you keep a full feeling longer.

- **Insoluble fibers** are not digested; so they act like brooms sweeping through your digestive system and ushering out those partially digested remnants from yesterday's meal. This type of fiber prevents constipation and improves a number of digestive problems such as spastic colon and hemorrhoids.

You should eat eight or nine servings of high fiber foods everyday. This isn't as tough as it seems if you eat your vegetables and fruits and choose whole grain breads and cereals. If you ever have colon polyps, you'll want to bump up the amount of fiber in your diet.

Building with proteins

Proteins help build and repair cells, muscles, and tissues.

Meat, fish, and dairy products, as well as peas and beans, are foods high in protein. Most of these foods, with the exception of peas and beans, also contain high levels of fat and cholesterol. (Chapter 5 tells you about the dangers of too much cholesterol).

So how do you keep your body healthy while getting adequate amounts of protein? By choosing lean cuts of meat over fatty cuts. Put fish or chicken on your plate more often than red meat. Place low-fat milk products in your grocery cart instead of their whole-milk cousins. And limit your daily calories from protein to 10 to 20 percent of your total intake.

Most Americans eat a lot more protein than they really need. You only need four ounces of protein per day. (A four-ounce serving of meat is about the size of a deck of cards.) A serving of fish or meat and a couple servings of low-fat dairy products will give you enough protein for the day.

Energizing with fats

Fats supply fatty acids that your body can't produce and help your body absorb the (fat-soluble) vitamins A, D, E, and K.

Per gram, fats give you twice the energy of carbohydrates and proteins, but they also contain *twice* the calories! High-fat foods are packed with calories and help you gain weight more quickly and easily than other foods. Fats also raise your cholesterol levels and increase your risk of cardiovascular disease, cancer, and diabetes.

You need a certain amount of fat in your diet, but you don't have to work to include it. Most Americans get way more fat than they need, which helps explain why the United States is an overweight nation.

Foods high in fats include both plant and animal foods. Here are just a few: fried foods, salad dressings, meats (bacon, roast beef, lamb, pork, hot dogs, and more), dairy products (cream cheese, butter, ice cream, cheese, milk, and so on), pastries, nuts, and many other foods we love! (For more info on the dangers of fats and cholesterol when it comes to your cardiovascular system, please check out Chapter 5.)

The lowdown on the three basic types of fats:

- ✔ **Saturated fats:** Found in butter, whole milk, meat, peanut butter, and pastries (among other things), saturated fats elevate your cholesterol and triglyceride levels.

  Avoid eating more than 10 to 20 milligrams of saturated fats a day (less if you can). _Trans-saturated fats_ ("trans fats") also raise cholesterol levels. You find these rascals in fried foods, bakery goods, and hard margarines. (Look for margarines that have "No trans fats" printed on their labels. Your heart will thank you.)

- ✔ **Polyunsaturated fats:** These fats usually come from plants. Corn oil, safflower oil, and many soft margarines fall into this category. Polyunsaturated fats lower your bad cholesterol (LDL), but they also lower your good cholesterol (HDL). Limit yourself to one tablespoon of polyunsaturated fats a day.

- ✔ **Monounsaturated fats:** Although these fats are a bit more helpful than the others, you still need to keep monounsaturated fats under control (between 15 and 25 milligrams per day, which equals about 2 tablespoons of oil). These fats lower your bad LDLs and keep your good HDLs high. You can find monounsaturated fats in peanuts and peanut oil, olives and olive oil, and avocados.

Opt for polyunsaturated and monounsaturated fats over saturated fats and trans fats. And take advantage of the low-fat options that line the aisles of grocery stores. If you keep your consumption of fats down, you can cut your risk of cancer.

Feeding flow

To maintain a high level of energy and keep yourself charging ahead throughout the day, you have to put the right type of fuel into your tanks and maintain a continuous flow of fuel to your body.

To maintain your energy level, build muscle, and burn calories, balance your eating over the course of the day. Eat at regular intervals — approximately every three to six hours. If you follow this timetable, snacks actually play a key role in your daylong meal plan. They add the right types of food for balance and keep you from feeling deprived of food. Make sure your snack is less than 150 calories.

Some people eat only once a day. Why? Some folks take up this bad habit in an attempt to lose weight. Others claim that they don't have time to eat throughout the day. Whatever the reason, it's a bad idea. If you only eat once a day, you're more likely to pig out when you do eat and get so stuffed that you feel tired and groggy after the meal. Plus, a once-a-day feeding regimen doesn't give your body the nutrients it needs to burn calories and build muscle and tissue throughout the day.

Meals on wheels

Most people don't want to carry around a food chart that lists the nutrients and calories in every possible food they may encounter throughout the day. The easiest way to plan and keep track of what you eat (without a chart) is to balance the portions of foods you put on your plate. A simple way to do that is to think of your plate as a wheel sectioned into quarters.

Put vegetables and fruit on half the wheel, place some form of protein (fish, meat, chicken,

beans, and so on) on one quarter of it, and reserve the other quarter for a starch (such as a whole-wheat roll or brown rice).

Worried that there's no fat on your wheel? Well, if you're like most folks and you put a bit of salad dressing on your salad (on the vegetable half of you plate) or margarine on your vegetable or roll, your meal already contains plenty of fat. Remember that a little bit of fat carries a lot of weight.

Eating to Prevent or Contain Problems

Feeding your body the right foods can help forestall some health problems and diet can be part of a treatment regimen for certain conditions. This section talks about the most helpful nutrients for health maintenance and prevention.

- **Antioxidants:** Ongoing research shows the importance of antioxidants in slowing the aging process. *Antioxidants* eliminate free radicals from your body. *Free radicals* are to your body what rust is to your car: They promote damage to your infrastructure, leading to heart disease, lower immunity, cataracts, diabetes, and cancer. Antioxidants hook up with the free radicals and escort them safely out of your body so they can do no harm. Colorful fruits and vegetables (such as broccoli, berries, grapes, and carrots) are especially high in antioxidants.

- **Fiber:** Fiber pushes food through your digestive system helping protect your body against colon cancer, *diverticulitis* (inflammation of the little pouches inside your colon), spastic colon, other digestive problems, and hemorrhoids. It helps lower your cholesterol levels and stabilizes blood-sugar levels. Fiber also gives you a full feeling and helps you control your weight.

  Fiber is found in the skins of vegetables and fruits and the outer layers of grains, so eating the skin of your baked potato and choosing whole grains helps increase the amount of fiber in your diet.

- **Soy:** Researchers are just beginning to discover the benefits of soy. It may protect against breast cancer, heart disease, and osteoporosis. Soy proteins and isoflavones are *phytoestrogens* (plant estrogens), which lower cholesterol and support your immune system. You can find soy in tofu, tempeh, soymilk, and soy yogurt.

A single serving of soy per day is beneficial. Some research indicates that too much soy can negatively impact your hormone balance.

Strengthening your bones

Osteoporosis (brittle bones) is particularly common in women after menopause because long periods of lower estrogen levels promote bone loss. To slow the rate of bone loss, it's important that you have plenty of calcium in your diet and an adequate supply of the vitamins that help your body absorb calcium.

Diet and exercise are two of the best and easiest ways to improve the health of your bones. In the following sections you'll find some great information for bone-healthy eating.

Feeding your calcium needs

You should ingest between 1,200 to 1,500 milligrams of calcium each day (check out the table in Chapter 4 for your exact dosage). If you want to break that down into an eating plan, you need to eat two cups of dairy products, one cup of juice with added calcium, and two calcium-rich foods each day.

Many foods are naturally high in calcium, including dairy products (try to get the low-fat type) and green leafy vegetables such as spinach and collard greens. Many juices and breakfast products (like cereal and frozen waffles) are "calcium-fortified," making it even easier to add calcium to your diet.

Many women don't get enough calcium through the foods they eat and find it easier to take calcium supplements. If you're one of these people, take supplements (usually a pill or chewable tablet) throughout the day rather than in one large dose. This way you'll ensure maximum absorption of the calcium.

Calcium citrate and *calcium carbonate* are the recommended supplements because they're more easily absorbed than calcium phosphate, calcium lactate, and calcium gluconate, and they're free from contaminants. Avoid using bone meal and dolomite as calcium supplements because they can be contaminated with lead.

Take calcium supplements with a glass of orange juice or tomato juice — the vitamin C helps you absorb the calcium. Taking calcium supplements with milk is also great because the lactose and vitamin D in milk also helps you absorb calcium.

Here are some great tips (if we do say so ourselves) to help you get more calcium into your diet:

✔ If you eat cereal for breakfast, try the brands that have 400 or 500 milligrams of calcium in each serving. Instant oatmeal is also a good source of calcium but only contains about 100 milligrams of calcium in each packet.

✔ Add low-fat grated cheese to baked potatoes, salads, toast, or your favorite vegetables.

✔ Combine fat-free ricotta cheese with fat-free cream cheese and a squeeze of honey for a great bagel spread. You get more calcium and a very satisfying treat.

✔ Add nonfat dry powdered milk to oatmeal, casseroles, pancakes, yogurt, or smoothies to bone up on calcium.

✔ Citrus juices with added vitamin D and calcium are easy to work into your daily routine and can give you much of the calcium you need each day.

✔ Some antacids not only relieve indigestion, they also contain 500 milligrams of calcium. They're worth a chew!

Absorbing some helper vitamins

You need 400 IU (international units) of vitamin D each day to help your body absorb calcium. That recommendation increases to 600 to 700 IU after your 70th birthday. But don't ever exceed 800 IU of vitamin D a day, because vitamin D is a fat-soluble vitamin and can be toxic if you get too much. Most milk products and cereals are fortified with vitamin D so it's not difficult to meet your daily requirements through a good breakfast.

You can get all the vitamin D you need by getting 10 to 15 minutes of sunshine each day. Sunshine stimulates your skin to produce vitamin D. (Take a walk and kill two birds with one stone! You can get your vitamin D *and* some exercise.)

Vitamin K is also good for your bones and is found in green vegetables such as lettuce, broccoli, cabbage, and spinach.

Potassium and magnesium are also critical in your quest to maintain bone strength. You can get these nutrients by including greens (as in collard greens, mustard greens and so forth), beans, whole grains, vegetables, and fruits in your meals every day.

Pumping up your cardiovascular system

Keeping your cardiovascular system healthy is a matter of keeping your blood lean and your vessels clean. Lean blood (low in LDL cholesterol — "bad cholesterol" — and triglycerides) prevents the fatty deposits that can lead to all sorts of cardiovascular problems from forming in your arteries.

Curbing the fats in your diet and replacing them with fruits, whole grains, and vegetables can help maintain healthy blood, arteries, and heart. The antioxidants, fiber, and other beneficial nutrients found in these plant foods help prevent cholesterol from oxidizing and damaging your arteries and heart.

Fruits and vegetables deliver more fiber and complex carbohydrates and less fat than any other food group, which is critical to maintaining lean and clean blood. Also, the calcium, antioxidants, and other vitamins found in fruits and vegetables keep your blood, blood vessels, and heart healthy. Plus fruits and vegetables are 90 percent water (low in calories) and very filling.

Watch those high-cholesterol foods like egg yolks, sausage, bacon, ice cream, butter, cheese, pastries, fried foods, and fatty cuts of meat. Not surprisingly, these foods can raise the cholesterol levels in your blood.

Watch your sodium if you're concerned about high blood pressure (and one out of five Americans should be concerned). Avoiding processed foods, smoked meats and fish, salty snack foods, canned vegetables, olives, pickles, and fast food can greatly reduce the sodium in your diet. Choose fresh vegetables and meats and low-sodium alternatives.

Weighing in on the Weight Issue

You know, we know, everybody knows that being overweight is unhealthy. We hate to tell you, but carrying excess weight around in your menopausal years carries even more health risks.

The good news is that menopause can provide the perfect opportunity to assess yourself and your goals near the midpoint of your life, and get you started down the road to a new, healthier you.

Realizing the perils of too much weight

Weight has an incredibly important effect on health. Overweight women are more likely to suffer heart disease, stroke, diabetes, and certain types of cancer. Overweight women are also more likely to die at a younger age than the average woman. Body fat (measured by your Body Mass Index — BMI — explained in the "Finding a healthy weight" sidebar) is an even better predictor of your potential for health problems than weight. Studies show that the higher your BMI, the greater your risk of hypertension (high blood pressure). Menopausal women are already more susceptible to hypertension and other cardiovascular diseases (see Chapter 5). So maintaining a healthy weight can help you keep your risk of cardiovascular problems as low as possible. Figure 18-1 can tell you where you fall in relation to the target weight for your height.

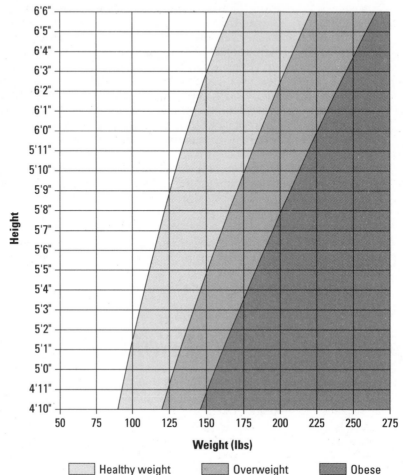

Figure 18-1:
Find out
where your
weight falls.

Extra weight not only collects around your middle after menopause, it also raises your risk for a variety of unhealthy conditions such as high cholesterol, *arteriosclerosis* (hardening of the arteries), heart disease, hypertension, diabetes, and stroke. Incidences of breast cancer, colon cancer, endometrial cancer, and gallstones also increase significantly in women who are overweight during and after menopause.

One of the best ways to help your overall quality of life during and after the change is to maintain a healthy weight.

The risk of hypertension begins to increase when your BMI gets above 20 and rises steadily as your BMI increases. It's thought that extra weight makes blood vessels constrict. Even a modest weight gain (five to ten pounds) after menopause raises your risk of *hypertension* (high blood pressure). A well-known study of thousands of nurses found that women who lost 10 to 20 pounds during the course of the study had a lower risk of hypertension than women who maintained a steady weight.

Because of estrogen's role in maintaining healthy blood and vessels, women's risk of cardiovascular problems rise after menopause as estrogen levels fall. In addition, your risk of cardiovascular disease increases even more as your BMI increases.

Adult-onset diabetes can lead to a slew of other medical conditions such as hypertension, circulation problems, skin ulcers, nerve disorders, stroke, blindness, heart disease, and kidney problems. If you've gained more than 12 pounds since you were 18, you've increased your risk of adult-onset diabetes; if you've gained more than 40 pounds, your risk of diabetes has gone way up, and you don't want that. Women who lose weight can reduce their risk of diabetes dramatically.

Finding a healthy weight

A *healthy weight* is one that is associated with people who have few health problems. You can find your recommended weight by referring to weight tables published by insurance companies. Insurance companies try to figure out the weight ranges for women who live the longest. This is one of the simplest ways to determine a healthy weight.

But your very own, personal healthy weight can be fine tuned by evaluating your body fat. Body fat is the real villain in this story, not weight. To measure body fat, visit your physician or health club. Your doc (or a helpful individual at your local club) will use calipers to measure the amount of fat in several places on your body, or if she wants to be really accurate, she'll immerse you in a tub of water to see how much water you displace. A good, general rule of thumb is that healthy women have between 18 and 27 percent body fat.

Another measurement, your *Body Mass Index* (BMI), is based on height and weight, provides a good estimation of body fat, and is easier to calculate. To determine your BMI:

1. Multiply your height (in inches) by itself

2. Divide your weight (in pounds) by the number you got in step 1.

3. Multiply your answer in step two by 705.

This is your BMI. If your score is under 25, you're in the healthy range. Women with a BMI over 30 (or if you're using a weight table — 20 percent over your recommended weight) are considered obese.

A quicker way to see if you're at a healthy weight is to look at Figure 18-1.

Eating to control body weight

Many of us struggle with controlling our weight, and it's no wonder. If you're like us, you grew up with a parent or grandparent telling you to "clean your plate if you want dessert" and with advertisements claiming that "nothin' says lovin' like somethin' from the oven!" But we're here to tell you that the struggle to control your weight is a worthwhile battle. Achieving or maintaining a healthy weight has a tremendous impact on your overall health.

You don't have to quit eating your favorite foods; just watch the size of your portions. Awareness is the first step.

Counting calories

To lose weight, you have to reduce the calories you eat and/or burn more calories through exercise. To maintain a healthy weight when you reach that point, you have to strike a balance between the calories you eat and the calories you burn through activity. But remember: You must get the proper nutrients to keep your body healthy and protect it from disease throughout the process. That's the secret to success.

Let's face it, nobody likes to count calories. If you're at a healthy weight and simply want to eat a healthier diet, just follow the advice in the "Meals on wheels" sidebar. You'll have more energy, suffer fewer food cravings, and help your body ward off disease and chronic medical conditions.

If your goal is to eat healthy to shed pounds, you need to become aware of the calories you're eating and the source of those calories. Keep your calories within a healthy range, add a bit of exercise five days a week, and you can shed pounds while you improve your health.

Most people can eliminate lots of empty calories — the calories you eat without a purpose just because they're there. Do you ever finish up the French fries on your child's plate? Do you snack on leftovers as you clear the table? If so, you're falling into the empty-calorie trap.

Here are the calorie recommendations for women:

- ✔ **To maintain your weight:** 1,500 to 1,600 calories a day
- ✔ **To lose weight:** 1,300 to 1,400 calories a day

If you're extremely active (exercising for more than an hour each day), add 100 calories to the recommendations.

Exercise burns up calories, so you can lose weight more easily and keep it off by incorporating exercise into your fitness plan. If some exercise tips sound like a good thing, check out Chapter 19.

If you're trying to watch your calories, watch the alcohol. Limit your alcohol intake to no more than three drinks (1½ ounces of liquor, a 4-ounce glass of wine, or 12 ounces of beer) a week. Wine and beer have about 100 to 150 calories. The alcohol in a mixed drink is 100 calories or so, and if you mix it with something sweet, you can consume up to 400 calories per drink.

Nibbling on little nothings

The following list provides some good nutritional tips that have little or no caloric cost:

✔ Lettuce, parsley, radishes, watercress, and celery provide nutrients without the calories.

✔ Use butter-flavored sprays when cooking instead of oil to shave off fat and calories.

✔ Sugar-free gelatin adds a bit of free dessert to any meal.

✔ Hot pepper and picante sauces add a bit of spice without a lot of calories.

✔ Low-fat bouillon is a great substitute for butter-based sauces when serving pasta or steamed vegetables.

✔ Fat-free cream cheese, mayonnaise, salad dressing, and sour cream are free in terms of fat calories as long as you use only 1 tablespoon.

Foregoing fat

It's really tough. Many of our favorite foods are high in fat. Take away the fat, and they don't seem so good. Believe it or not, we have some tips for eating *satisfying* meals that are a bit less fatty. If you really dislike the low-fat alternatives, go ahead and have the high-fat food, just reduce the portion size. Only eat half of that bratwurst or eat a donut hole instead of the whole donut. Here are some other great tips:

✔ Try mixing instant bouillon in hot water and adding a few tablespoons to vegetables, rice, or pasta instead of putting butter or margarine on the food. You get that rich taste without the fat.

✔ Choose lean cuts of beef (tenderloin instead of rib-eye, for example) — they have less marbling than the fattier cuts.

✔ Try putting low-fat yogurt or low-fat cottage cheese on top of your baked potato instead of butter or sour cream.

✔ When you order a salad at a restaurant, get the salad dressing on the side. And, if the restaurant doesn't have a low-fat alternative, try using one tablespoon of a vinaigrette.

✔ Eat spicy toppings like salsa, ginger, or picante sauce instead of cream sauces.

Discouraging diets

It seems as if someone is always pushing a new diet that promises to make weight disappear using a secret no one else has discovered. Many of us try one of these "miracle" diets and end up looking for a new one because the weight we lose reappears. The secret to getting to a healthy weight and staying there is to — are you ready for this? — avoid diets. Most diets have you chomping at the bit, waiting for the pounds to come off so you can go back to eating the foods you want. When you go back to your old habits, the weight returns.

Eating healthier can help you lose weight and keep it off because it encourages you to change the way you think about food. You begin to think about food as a fuel, as opposed to a treat that you can't have or a substance that you must eat despite its cardboard-like flavor. You begin to think about what your body needs to stay lean, build muscle, rejuvenate tissue, and ward off disease.

Beware of unbalanced diets that tell you to completely avoid one of the major nutrients (complex carbohydrates, fats, or protein). By cutting out one of these groups, you may also eliminate fiber, antioxidants, or phytochemicals that protect your body from aging and disease.

Low-carbohydrate and high-protein diets are high in cholesterol and low in fiber, which may increase your risk of heart disease, cancer, and digestive problems.

Liquid diets offer quick weight loss, but you mostly lose muscle. When you lose more muscle than fat, you actually have a higher percent of body fat even though you weigh less. Also, some liquid diets can damage your heart, kidney, and liver and cause an irregular heartbeat and many other health problems.

Chapter 19

Focusing on Fitness

With all the changes going on with your body, now is a great time to make sure that you're physically fit. Physical activity and exercise during perimenopause and menopause can relieve many of the common physical and mental/emotional symptoms that accompany the change.

We have some good news: You don't need to be an athlete or join a health club to realize tremendous health benefits from exercise. According to several studies, one hour of moderate exercise five times a week improves the quality and quantity of your life. In this chapter, we introduce you to exercises that you can do in your home and ways to fit fitness into an already busy life.

Maybe you're already physically active, and you want to move your program up a notch. If so, you're in the healthy minority. Studies indicate that only 20 percent of American women get 30 minutes of exercise five times a week. We don't forget about you in this chapter just because you have a head start on some other women. We offer plenty of tips for everyone. You can see how your current fitness program reduces your risk for many medical conditions and find some suggestions to help you vary or supplement your routine.

Benefiting from Exercise during the Menopausal Years

The lower estrogen levels in your body during the change can contribute to a number of medical conditions, memory lapses, and emotional transformations. Physical activity can help you reclaim your grip on life and fight off cardiovascular disease, diabetes, cancer, osteoporosis, and more.

The type of physical activity we're talking about consists of movement that burns calories. Jogging or playing tennis burns lots of calories quickly, but seemingly mundane activities like vacuuming, gardening, and raking leaves can be beneficial if you do them for a long enough period of time (45 minutes to an hour). The trade-off is simple: Do a vigorous activity for a short period of time or a moderately demanding activity for a longer period of time.

Many terrific studies show that physical activity makes a difference in the health of menopausal women. Exercise puts a positive spin on many of the health concerns women face during and after the change.

Tweaking your attitude

A variety of studies show that exercise and physical activity improve your ability to cope with stress and depression. One study even shows that running is more effective than psychotherapy for reducing depression, and the results aren't that difficult to believe. The term *runner's high* isn't a joke — physical activity helps your body release *endorphins,* substances that naturally relieve pain and elevate your mood.

You can relieve the perimenopausal symptoms of anxiety, irritability, mood swings, decreased libido, and depression by sticking to a fitness plan that gives you time to build your mental and physical fitness.

Setting aside some time for exercise each day also helps you organize your thoughts and feelings, relieve stress and anxiety, and re-establish your grip on life. If you make the initial effort, you'll begin to look forward to *your* time.

Flushing less; sleeping more

Only about 1 in 20 women who exercise experience hot flashes. Compare that stat to the ratio of women in the non-exercising crowd who experience hot flashes — about 1 in 4 — and you can quickly see why tying on those sneakers and going for a walk is a good thing. Hot flashes are a pain in their own right, but they can also turn into night sweats and cost you precious dream time. Exercise can lessen this effect and make your sleep more restful.

Exercise also helps women sleep better at night for another reason. Yes, exercise makes you tired, but there's more to the story. Exercise affects the amount of *melatonin* (a hormone that helps regulate sleep) in your body.

Melatonin levels are normally high in young children, but they appear to decline gradually with age in some adults. Exercise keeps the pineal gland producing melatonin at night (when levels are naturally higher), even though melatonin levels actually decline when you exercise.

Shedding pounds

Women typically gain about one pound a year from their late thirties through their mid-sixties. A pound may not sound like much, but it adds up over the years. Weight gain raises your risk of many diseases. Women who incorporate 20 to 30 minutes of physical activity into their lives *every day* can maintain their present weight or lose weight (but exercising an hour each day is the prescription for overall health).

You can find all kinds of ways to lose weight, but to lose weight and keep it off, walking is one of the most effective physical activities. After studying thousands of dieters, one study found that 49 out of 50 people who lost 30 pounds or more walked for at least half an hour at a brisk pace every day. The bonus: You don't need any equipment or special conditions other than comfortable shoes and personal motivation.

Keeping your heart healthy

Just because a woman generally has the heart of a man ten years her junior because of the estrogen her body produces, doesn't mean that heart disease doesn't catch up with the female of the species. Keeping your heart healthy through diet, exercise, and medication, if necessary, should be a priority for your menopausal years.

Cleaning up with good cholesterol levels

Physically active women tend to have higher levels of the good cholesterol (HDL) than women who aren't so active. If you start exercising today, you can notice better HDL-cholesterol levels within a few months. Regular exercise also prevents the bad cholesterol (LDL) from building up and clogging your arteries.

Listening to a beating heart

Because physical activity improves your cholesterol profile, your blood vessels are less apt to play host to fatty buildup that results in arteriosclerosis. Arteriosclerosis can cause hypertension (high blood pressure), heart disease, and stroke, so getting physical reduces your risk of all three.

A very famous study (the Nurses' Health Study) revealed that walking briskly for three hours a week can reduce your risk of heart disease by 40 to 50 percent. The study also showed that even women who just started walking regularly benefited by reducing their risk of heart disease.

The more often you exercise and the longer your workout, the more benefits you gain.

Keeping a lid on blood pressure

Because exercise improves your cholesterol profile, your risk of high blood pressure goes down too. With a healthier cholesterol profile, your blood vessels are less likely to get clogged with *plaque* (deposits of fat mixed with other substances that are covered with a layer of calcium and found on the walls of your blood vessels). Arteriosclerosis causes your blood vessels to narrow and forces your heart to beat harder to get the blood through, raising the pressure in your blood vessels and resulting in hypertension (high blood pressure).

Exercising sound judgment

In case you haven't guessed by now, regular exercise seems to cure whatever ails you. This statement is especially true in relation to cardiovascular disease. Moderate exercise, such as walking for 30 minutes five times a week, can improve the health of your body and mind.

Exercise benefits your cardiovascular system in many ways:

- ✔ Improves your circulation
- ✔ Increases your good (HDL) cholesterol levels
- ✔ Reduces total cholesterol, triglycerides, and blood pressure
- ✔ Increases your endurance
- ✔ Reduces anxiety, depression, and emotional stress
- ✔ Builds another support group when you do it with friends

Shoring up your bones

After menopause, women begin losing bone density. They risk developing *osteoporosis* (brittle bones; check out Chapter 4 for more info) as a result of the loss. People who have osteoporosis are prone to fractures. This tendency forces them to restrict their daily activity, which in turn impacts the quality and longevity of their life.

To prevent osteoporosis and fractures, take our advice:

- ✔ Include weight-bearing exercises in your exercise routines to increase bone density (bone strength) and to slow or prevent bone loss. (See "Strengthening bones and toning muscle" later in this chapter.)
- ✔ Improve your balance and flexibility with exercise that can help you reduce your risk of falling and fracturing your bones. (Jump to the "Flexing through stretching" section later on for more information.)

Doing without diabetes

Diabetes is a serious health condition that can produce a host of other medical problems ranging from hypertension to blindness. Exercise can reduce your risk of adult-onset diabetes by helping you keep your weight in a safe range and by improving your body's response to insulin. (For more on diabetes, see Chapter 14.)

Even if you're overweight or leading a sedentary lifestyle now, you can reduce your risk of becoming diabetic by beginning a fitness program. A small increase in activity will help, but more activity provides more protection from developing diabetes. In one study, women who walked briskly for three hours a week reduced their risk of diabetes as much as women who worked out vigorously for half that amount of time. Our point? You don't need to train for a marathon to reduce your risk of diabetes.

Steering clear of colon cancer

In Chapter 13 we discuss the benefits of getting your colon checked regularly. Exercise is another way to protect yourself against colon cancer. Exercise keeps waste (and any carcinogens you may have ingested) moving through your digestive tract and out of your body so the waste doesn't linger in your colon. The level of activity we recommend earlier in this chapter (an hour a day five days a week) offers some protection against colon cancer.

Sharpening your memory

Staying active as you age is proven to have a very positive impact on memory and judgment. Getting more blood and oxygen flowing to your brain seems to trigger these positive effects.

Living long and prospering

Without cracking open a fortune cookie, we can say with some confidence that daily exercise can extend your life. One group of 60- to 80-year-olds cut their death rate in half by walking two miles every day. Not too shabby.

Focusing on the Fundamental Facets of Fitness

Whatever activities you decide to do to improve your physical fitness, make sure that you enjoy them. If you don't like an activity, you won't work it into your daily schedule, and you won't do it for long.

Plan your week out in advance to make sure that you reserve time for your workout. Make your fitness time a priority that you won't give it up whenever things get busy. Working physical activity into your day helps you accomplish your primary long-term goal — living a long and healthy life — and it makes you feel pretty good in the short term too.

Getting started

If you haven't been getting much exercise, begin your program slowly. For the first few weeks, exercise three times a week for about 20 or 30 minutes per session. Then, when you feel good with that pace and decide you want to bump it up a notch, add a few more days and a little more time to your workout. Another way to move to the next level is to increase the intensity of your workout. If you're walking, go further or faster or walk twice a day on certain days of the week. Or you may want to start jogging instead of walking. The bottom line: You gain more by exercising longer or faster.

Regardless of how you decide to increase the intensity of your workout, make sure that your body gets used to each level before you move on to the next. If you start experiencing any abnormal symptoms (such as chest pain, shortness of breath, and so on) as you increase your exercise intensity, please see your doctor.

Health clubs or the local YMCA are nice because they offer motivation and instruction as well as an opportunity to form a support group with people who are also trying to stay healthy. But you don't have to join a club to receive these kinds of benefits. Asking a friend from your neighborhood to join in your morning walk or play a set of tennis can also provide the support and motivation you need to stick with it.

If you have any health problems, visit your doctor for a thorough physical before starting a new or more vigorous exercise program.

Fitting in fitness

Does anyone have a spare hour (or half-hour) in his or her day? When someone raises the subject of exercise, many women think, "I don't have time to take a walk or work out." We know that taking care of the approximately 12 million errands that your children, spouse, parents, and friends approach you with every day leaves you with little discretionary time or energy.

But fitness time is time that you devote to your health. Your family and your friends would agree that nothing is more important than your health. Besides, you're going to take time out of your life and away from your family and friends for your health whether you exercise or not. So, either take the time to exercise now or spend some time with the medical professionals taking care of your health later.

Here are five simple ways you can incorporate physical activity into an already busy day.

1. Take the stairs instead of the elevator. Whether you go up or down, you get your blood pumping and your legs working.

2. When you're talking on the phone, stand up and stretch. Put your foot up on the table and stretch your hamstrings, do a few squats, bend from side to side, or walk around.

3. When you go shopping, park your car away from the store and walk briskly to your destination. When you're in a mall, take a lap or two (who knows, you may spot a sale).

4. Make a permanent appointment with yourself to take a brisk walk first thing in the morning or after dinner each day — and make this the most important appointment of your day.

A walk first thing in the morning can help you organize your day. An after-dinner walk can help you wind down from a busy day so that you sleep better. Remember, this is time you devote to keeping yourself healthy so your loved ones can hang onto you longer.

5. Use your lunch hour or break time at work to climb the stairs or take a walk around the building. On days when you can't get any other exercise, this may be the only time you have to get moving. Remember: Every little bit helps.

Planning your program

After the onset of perimenopause, you want to keep your hormones balanced, your diet balanced, and yes, your fitness program balanced. You should incorporate three types of activities into your fitness routine: aerobic exercise, flexibility training, and strength training. You're probably wondering how long this workout is going to take. Don't worry — you don't have to do all three each day, but you should fit all three in your weekly fitness plan.

✔ **Aerobic activity:** This form of exercise is great for your cardiovascular system. Aerobic activity helps your endurance, but it also helps you burn fat. Basically, it's the perfect type of exercise for women of all ages. Whether you perform your aerobic activities in vigorous, relatively short bursts or at a slightly slower pace for longer periods of time, the benefits work out the same. For example, you can burn 200 calories by walking for 30 minutes or by jogging for 18 minutes.

Aerobic exercise benefits your body because it forces your cardiovascular system and muscles to exert themselves. Too little exertion, and you don't gain all the benefits of exercise; too much exertion, and you stress your cardiovascular system (and your muscles).

More vigorous forms of aerobic exercise include jogging, walking, cycling, aerobic dance, martial arts, and jumping rope. Even activities you probably don't think of as exercise can give you a light aerobic workout — walking your dog, golfing, shopping, gardening, or playing with the kids.

✔ **Flexibility training:** This aspect of your workout routine can protect you from injury, improve your balance, and provide muscle flexibility. Stretching is the simplest and easiest way to improve your flexibility and agility. Working with a *Swiss ball* (a colorful exercise ball you can find in health clubs that are anywhere from two to three feet in diameter) can improve your flexibility and balance while strengthening and toning your muscles. Yoga is probably the oldest form of stretching.

✔ **Strength training:** Incorporating strength training into your exercise schedule helps you build muscle tone, endurance, and bone density. Because strength training builds muscle, it speeds up your metabolism so you burn more calories — even when you're resting. (Muscle burns more calories than fat does, so the more muscle you have, the more calories you burn.)

Scheduling fitness fun time

A total fitness program incorporates aerobic exercise, flexibility training, and strength training in a weekly fitness plan. In this section, we provide an example of a balanced program, incorporating all three training elements.

Basically the plan includes two rest days each week (preferably not back to back) and one easy day. On the other days, you should give it your best — work out at a comfortable but challenging pace. Breaking your workout into two or three sessions during the day because of time constraints is fine. And you can modify your days to suit your personal preferences.

Be sure to warm up before each session and cool down afterwards. (For more information, see the "Warming up and cooling down" section in this chapter.) In the fitness programs mentioned here, we fit stretching into the program by doing it as part of our warm-up and cool-down routines, but you can add more stretching to your program or add a yoga class to your schedule. Stretching improves flexibility and keeps your muscles from getting sore.

Start your fitness calendar on whatever day of the week makes sense to you. Many people start it on Monday to coincide with the workweek. Doing so with the routine we outline lets you start your week with a good workout and end it with a rest day. Or maybe you're the type of person who prefers to start your week slowly and increase your level of activity as you go. You decide.

✔ **Day 1:** We assume that you like to hit each new week running, so start Day 1 off with a warm-up. Then move onto 20 to 30 minutes of aerobic activity followed by 20 minutes of strength training (see the "Strengthening bones and toning muscle" section later in this chapter). End your workout with a cool-down that includes at least 5 to 10 minutes of stretching.

✔ **Day 2:** Do 20 to 30 minutes of aerobic exercise but at a lower intensity than your Day 1 workout. Remember your warm-up and cool-down time.

✔ **Day 3:** Do the Day 1 routine — warm-up, aerobic exercise, strength training, and then a cool-down with some good stretching. Your intensity should be the same as that of Day 1.

✔ **Day 4:** Take a day off to rest and restore your muscles. Resting is also important for your body.

✔ **Day 5:** Follow the same workout as Days 1 and 3.

✔ **Day 6:** This is ladies' choice day. Do something different for your aerobic exercise, something a bit lighter — gardening, dancing, yard work, swimming with the kids, or golfing — but do it for 45 minutes rather than a half-hour.

✔ **Day 7:** Take the day to rest and relax to restore your muscles.

Getting Personal about Your Fitness Plan

Planning is essential to doing. If you don't have a plan, making something happen and tracking your progress is hard. You begin slowly and work your way up to more intense, more frequent, and longer lasting workouts. You can also incorporate some of the strength-training and flexibility-training exercises into your weekly workout.

If you haven't exercised in a long time, you have heart disease, you're overweight, or you have any other medical condition, talk to your doctor about your fitness plan or find a certified personal trainer to guide you.

Zoning in on your target heart rate

The best way to make sure you're doing enough exercise to benefit your health and your heart is to check your *heart rate* (how fast your heart is beating). Your heart rate tells you how much effort you put into an exercise. Here's how you can check your heart rate:

1. Put your index and middle finger on your opposite wrist and find your pulse. (You can also use the carotid artery in your neck, which is under your jawbone.)

2. Count the number of beats for ten seconds (you need a clock with a second hand).

3. Multiply that number (the number of beats in ten seconds) by six. The result is your number of heart beats per minute — your heart rate.

After you know how to figure out your heart rate, you can figure out your *target heart-rate zone,* which is important when exercising. You should try to keep your heart rate within your target heart-rate zone during exercise to achieve the perfect workout intensity and maximum benefits.

1. Subtract your age from 220, which is the maximum heart rate (a heart rate you don't want to even approach).

2. Multiply your answer from Step 1 by 0.6. The resulting number is the lower limit of your target heart-rate zone.

3. Multiply your answer from Step 1 by 0.85. The resulting number is the upper limit of your target heart-rate zone.

Flexing through stretching

What's so tough about stretching? You probably did it back when you were taking grade-school gym class, doing ballet, or running track, right? Well, things have changed a bit. In the past few years, medical and exercise experts have come a long way in understanding the physics behind stretching. Some of the old stretching exercises actually hurt your body more than they helped it. So read on for some good advice about stretching. (And check out Figures 19-1 through 19-6 in the next section for a great introductory stretching routine.)

✔ Don't bounce. Stretch slowly until you feel some tension, not pain.

✔ When warming up, hold the position for 10 to 30 seconds, relax, and then stretch again.

✔ When cooling down, hold the position 30 seconds, relax, and then stretch again. If you're working on flexibility, try doing each stretch twice during the cool-down and stretch a bit further the second time.

If you increase your stretching intensity during the cool-down period when your muscles are already warm, you can increase your range of motion and get more out of your stretch. Stretching when your muscles are warm helps you build flexibility much more quickly because warm muscles stretch better than cold ones, and elastic and stretched muscles are flexible muscles.

✔ Never stretch a muscle if you've had a recent muscle, ligament, tendon, joint, or bone injury or if you feel a sharp pain. If you feel a sharp pain — as opposed to the dull ache of well-exercised muscles — consult your doctor before continuing with your stretching routine.

If you're interested in additional information on stretching, take a look at the resources in Appendix B.

Yoga is a terrific activity if you really want to work on your flexibility and balance. Yoga consists of three main components: exercise, breathing, and meditation. Over a hundred different schools of yoga exist, so find the form that suits your objectives. Like any physical workout, begin slowly and be patient with yourself. If you're interested in finding out more about yoga, check out the Web site of the American Yoga Association at www.american yogaassociation.org or check out *Power Yoga For Dummies* (Doug Swenson, Wiley Publishing, Inc.).

Warming up and cooling down

Be sure to start *each workout* with an easy warm-up period and end each session with a cool-down period. Warming up puts your muscles and cardio-vascular system on alert that they're about to go to work. Cooling down gives them a chance to relax after a satisfying workout. You can do the same activities for both your warm-up and cool-down sessions.

Warming up and cooling down can be as simple as walking or cycling for four or five minutes and then doing some *light, gentle* stretching for another five minutes.

Never stretch cold muscles — you can damage them. That's why you start your warm-up session with a bit of walking or cycling. Also, don't bounce or pull hard as you stretch during your warm-up, a time when your muscles are still pretty cold.

If you're worried about time, you may be inclined to skip your warm-up and jump right into your routine. Not a good idea. Warming up prevents injury and helps you ease into your workout without straining your muscles. Starting slowly actually lets you exercise longer.

The six simple stretches shown in Figures 19-1 through 19-6 stretch each of your major muscle groups. Try holding each stretch for 10 to 30 seconds. Over time, you may want to try to stretch further, which is great, but don't strain your muscles and be sure to stop when you feel tightness — don't stretch until you feel pain. If you stretch until you hurt, your muscles actually begin to contract, and you don't accomplish anything except hurting your muscles.

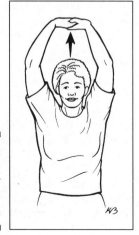

Figure 19-1:
Stretching
your upper
torso and
arms.

1. Clasp your hands above your head, interlocking your fingers.

2. Push your palms upward.

3. Stretch until you feel tightness and hold.

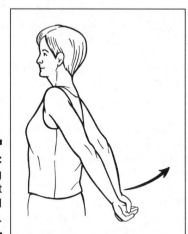

Figure 19-2:
Stretching
your chest
and
shoulders.

1. Clasp you hands behind your back.

2. Slowly and carefully lift your arms.

3. Stretch until you feel tightness and hold.

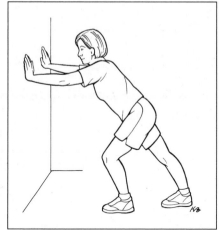

Figure 19-3:
Stretching
your
legs — all
the way.

1. Stand close to a wall with one leg forward.

2. Bend your front leg at the knee and keep your back leg straight.

3. Steady yourself by putting your hands on the wall.

4. Stretch forward keeping your back foot (including your heel) flat on the floor.

5. Switch legs and repeat Steps 1 through 4.

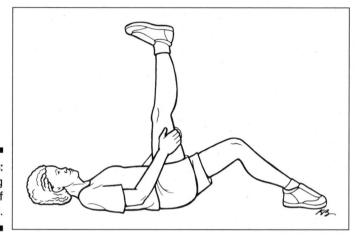

Figure 19-4:
Stretching
more of
your legs.

1. Lie flat on your back.

2. Stick one leg up in the air.

3. Grab your thigh below your knee.

4. Slightly bend the leg that is on the floor at the knee.

5. Gently pull your leg toward your chest keeping this leg straight.

6. Repeat Steps 1 though 5 with the opposite leg.

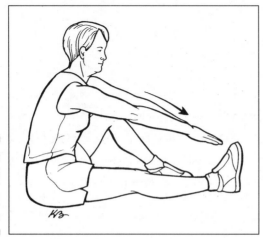

Figure 19-5:
Stretching
your lower
back and
buttocks.

1. Sit on the floor with both legs extended straight out in front of you.

2. Bend one leg so that your knee touches your chest.

3. Lean forward, reach out, and touch your toes.

   If you can't touch your toes, stretch as far as possible without experiencing pain. With time, you'll be able to get closer and closer.

4. Repeat Steps 1 through 3 with the opposite leg.

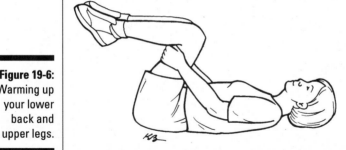

Figure 19-6:
Warming up
your lower
back and
upper legs.

1. Lie on your back.

2. Raise your legs in the air and bend them at the knee.

3. Grab both legs behind and below the knee.

4. While keeping your back as flat to the floor as possible, pull your thighs in toward your chest.

 A lot of people tend to cheat at the end of their workout, but definitely do some light stretching as part of your cool-down — it's terrific for your flexibility. You can stretch further and more easily after your muscles are really warm from prolonged exercise. You can make great strides in your flexibility and agility by doing five or ten minutes of stretching after your workout.

Exercises for Women with Osteoporosis

The best exercises to prevent or slow down osteoporosis are *weight-bearing exercises* — exercises, such as walking and strength training, that include gravity and tension on your muscles. Stress builds bone (see, stress is good for something), and putting weight on your bones provides the stress your bones need to grow in strength. Weight-bearing exercise promotes bone growth, which is critical for women of any age. During and after the change, when your estrogen levels are lower, weight-bearing exercise can keep bones strong and healthy by increasing bone density.

Although you move your muscles when you swim or cycle, these aren't the best exercises for building bone. The water (in swimming) and the bicycle seat (in cycling) take a lot of the load off your bones.

If you have osteoporosis, your bones may be more liable to break. Weight-bearing exercises are great for strengthening bone, but increasing your flexibility and balance can also help you avoid osteoporosis-related complications by reducing your risk of falling and breaking bones in the first place. You can improve your flexibility by including stretching in your fitness routine. (check out the two preceding sections) And you can improve your balance through exercise as well.

In the following sections, we discuss strength-training and balance exercises — two types of exercise that can help you fight osteoporosis and osteoporosis-related complications when incorporated into your fitness program. (For more information on walking, another weight-bearing exercise that, like strength training, can help you build bone, check out the "Walking for fun and fitness" section later in this chapter.)

Strengthening bones and toning muscle

Walking is a great way to fight osteoporosis, but a combination of walking and strength training is even better for building bone. You may choose to do both of these weight-bearing exercise routines on the same day or split them up during the course of the week — whatever your schedule allows. Weight-bearing exercises strengthen only the bones that you work, so walking strengthens your legs, but it won't help your other bones. You need to introduce strength-training exercises into your fitness program to accomplish that feat.

The best strength-training program is one that includes all your major muscle groups. This type of program improves your bone density in important areas, but it also improves your balance, which is important in avoiding falls that can cause fractures.

Start your strength-training regimen with a good, all-around strength-training routine using the seven exercises shown in Figures 19-7 through 19-13. These exercises strengthen your chest, arm, shoulder, leg, abdominal, and back muscles. You can start with 3 to 5 repetitions of each exercise and increase the number as your interest and endurance dictates. If you want to vary this routine or try some more advanced strength-training exercises, check out Appendix B for additional resources.

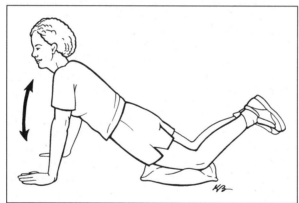

Figure 19-7:
Push-ups
for
beginners.

1. Kneel on the floor.

2. Place your hands a little wider than shoulder-width apart on the floor in front of you.

3. Keeping your knees on the floor (or on a cushion on the floor), raise your feet a bit.

4. Lower your upper body by bending your elbows.

5. Push back up and straighten your elbows.

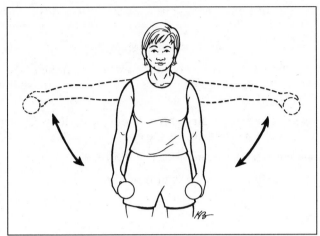

Figure 19-8:
Lateral
raises.

1. Stand up straight with your chest out and knees slightly bent.

2. Hold a two-pound weight in each hand with your arms down at your side.

3. With your elbows slightly bent, raise your hands to shoulder level. (Don't raise them higher than shoulder level.)

4. Slowly lower your hands until the weights are back at your side.

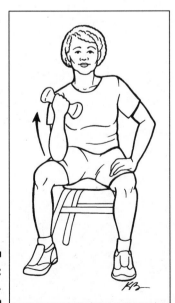

Figure 19-9:
Bicep curls.

1. Sit on the edge of a chair with your back straight and your legs slightly apart.

2. Lean forward (keeping your back straight).

3. Bend your elbow toward your chest and place it on the corresponding thigh while holding a two-pound weight. (You can increase the weight as you get stronger.)

4. Slowly lower your arm by straightening out your elbow. (The palm of your hand should be facing up at the end of the motion.)

5. Bring the weight back toward your chest.

6. Repeat Steps 1 through 5 with your other arm.

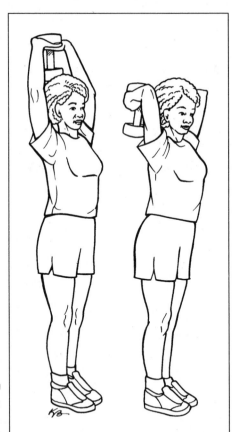

Figure 19-10:
Tricep curls.

1. Stand up straight with your knees bent slightly.

2. Hold a two-pound weight with both hands and raise it over your head.

3. Keeping your arms close to your head, lower the weight behind your head by bending your elbows.

4. When your forearm touches your upper arm, slowly raise the weight back up.

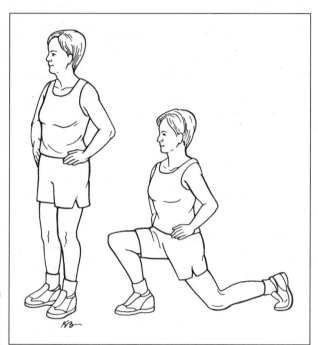

Figure 19-11:
Lunges.

1. Stand up straight with your hands on your hips.

2. Step forward with your right leg, keeping your back, neck, and head straight.

3. As your front heel hits the ground, bend both knees so that your left knee almost touches the floor (or go as low as you can).

4. Step back to the starting position.

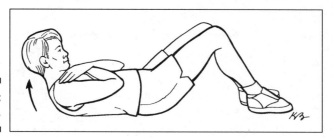

Figure 19-12:
Crunches.

1. Lie on your back with your arms crossed over your chest and both legs bent so that your shoes rest flat on the floor.

2. Slowly lift your upper body until your back is flat on the floor.

   Don't just lift your head or you'll exercise your neck instead of your abdomen. And don't strain to pull your upper body further up — just pull until your back is flat on the floor.

3. Relax and slowly lower yourself back to the floor.

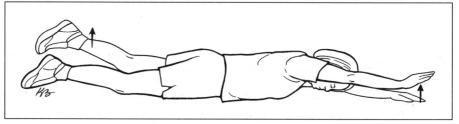

Figure 19-13:
Back
extensions.

1. Lie face down on the floor with both legs straight out behind you and both arms straight out over your head with your palms facing down.

2. Keeping your knees and elbows as straight as you can and your hips, tummy, and forehead flat on the floor, slowly lift your right arm and your left leg at the same time.

   Don't laugh. It's not as easy as you may think.

3. Switch sides and lift your left arm and right leg at the same time.

Adding balance to your routine

To avoid falling and possibly breaking a bone, spend some time working on balance. You can challenge the muscles that keep you balanced in many fun ways, and you can tone your muscles at the same time. Talk to a personal trainer to find out more about the following exercise aids:

✔ **Fitness balls:** Sometimes called Swiss balls or exercise balls, fitness balls are becoming very popular because they help you strengthen the *core balancing muscles* (abdominal, back, and hip muscles) that you use in many everyday activities.

If you're up for a challenge, sit on one of these balls and try to lift your feet; you can work up a sweat, exercise your abdominal muscles, and feel like a seal in a sideshow all at the same time. There are a million ways to use these balls to improve your balance, as well as your muscle tone.

✔ **Balance boards:** Stepping on this board feels like jumping on a moving surfboard after drinking three glasses of wine. Essentially, a ball is attached to the bottom of the board to challenge your balance (to say the least). As you strengthen your "balance" muscles with this contraption, you improve your overall sense of balance and your muscle tone.

✔ **Exercise tubing:** If your friends or family members see you with this one, they'll think that you're playing with a giant rubber band, so you may want to use this exercise aid in private. Exercise tubing is used in conjunction with stretching to increase flexibility.

All of these props can help you improve your balance, flexibility, and strength. They can be used at home or in the health club.

Exercises to Protect Your Heart

A balanced fitness plan will keep you healthy after menopause. The aerobic exercises are perfect for reducing your risk of hypertension, heart disease, stroke, arteriosclerosis, and other types of cardiovascular disease. These exercises, which are the core of a good cardiovascular workout, increase your blood circulation, strengthen your heart muscles, and improve your cholesterol profile.

Working on and working up to heart health

You can choose from any number of great aerobic sports or activities to improve your fitness. Cycling, jogging, swimming, and stair climbing are few examples. If you want to vary your workout, try an aerobic activity other than walking or check out the resources in Appendix B that have more info on beginning a fitness plan.

In the following "Walking for fun and fitness" section, we outline a walking regimen, which is an excellent way to begin your cardiovascular workout.

Incorporating stretching and strength training into your aerobic workout provides some variety to keep things fun (and ensures that you don't quit your aerobic routine because it becomes monotonous), increases your cardiovascular endurance, and allows you to quicken your pace. Try to work your way up to a routine similar to the one we lay out in the "Scheduling fitness fun time" section earlier in this chapter.

As you improve your cardiovascular fitness, you'll feel less tired when you workout even though you're doing the same amount of exercise. You'll also notice that your heart rate will gradually decrease, both during exercise and when at rest.

Build your endurance and stamina slowly. Don't over do it when you first begin an exercise program. Be sure to stay within your *target heart range* (see the "Zoning in on your target heart rate" sidebar in this chapter). If you're a beginner, keep to the lower end of your target range until you establish a comfortable workout plan. You can lower your risk of heart problems associated with exercise if you monitor your heart rate. To get the most out of your aerobic exercise, exercise at your target heart rate for at least 20 minutes.

A simple way to check whether your workout intensity is appropriate is what we call the *walk-and-talk test.* If you're exerting yourself but you can still carry on a conversation while you exercise, you're probably exercising at the right pace.

Exercise is the best gift you can give your cardiovascular system. Just 30 minutes of walking five or more times a week can effectively improve your cardiovascular health. All you need for walking is a comfortable pair of shoes and 30 minutes. If you need to break your workout up into two 15-minute sessions or three 10-minute sessions during the day, don't worry; it still works!

If you want to continue to build your cardiovascular fitness, increase the intensity of your workout by increasing the

- Distance.
- Speed.
- Time you spend doing the activity.
- Number of days you exercise.
- Level of difficulty of your course. (If you're a walker or cyclist, find a hilly course; if you use a treadmill, increase the incline or spend some time on a stair-climbing machine.)

As you increase the intensity of your workout, your cardiovascular fitness will improve and you will burn more calories. But, when you make your workout more challenging, do it slowly and take one step at a time. For example, you may choose to exercise at the same pace but add another ½ mile to your walk. Try the new distance out for a few weeks to make sure you're not going to be sore.

Walking for fun and fitness

As an exercise of choice, walking is perhaps the easiest way to begin a fitness program. You don't need a bunch of equipment; all you need is the will to get moving. But before you put your feet to the pavement, you have to map out a route you'll follow on you daily trek. Here are some pointers:

✔ Measure out a 2-mile course that you can easily expand to a 3-mile course when you want to increase the length of your walk.

✔ Pick a pretty area in your neighborhood, around your workplace, or at a local park. Or maybe your neighborhood park or school has a track you can use (though circling a track can get monotonous).

✔ Make sure that your route is conveniently located. You don't want to give yourself the "it takes too long to get there" excuse.

For the first two weeks of your new walking regimen, walk the 2 miles three times a week and time yourself. Your pace should be brisk enough to get your heart pumping, but not too fast that you can't talk and breathe at the same time. A good pace for many folks is to walk 2 miles in about 35 minutes. During Weeks 3 and 4, you can step up your program a bit. Walk four times a week instead of three. And try to increase your pace — do your 2 miles in a half-hour.

At this point in your exercise progression, you need to check yourself and see how you feel. How easy was the transition from Weeks 1 and 2 to Weeks 3 and 4? Do you feel like you can do more or are you comfortable with your current routine? Depending on your age and your health, you may want to stick with this walking schedule for a while. When you feel your body getting stronger and your outlook is ready for another challenge, you can move along to the next level. (For the sake of simplicity, we use a weekly progression to outline this entire schedule. But remember that your Week 5 doesn't have to begin until your ready for it.)

During the course of the next four weeks, your goal should be to walk 3 miles five times a week. Work up to this goal slowly. Add ½ mile to your distance during Week 5. At that point you're walking 2.5 miles four times during the week. Then, for Week 6, walk 2.5 miles again but try to walk five times this week instead of four times. Keep your pace brisk.

If you're ready to go on after Week 6, charge ahead and add another half mile to your distance and walk five times this week. By Weeks 7 and 8, you've reached your goal of walking 3 miles five times a week. But just because you've reached this goal doesn't mean you can't aim higher. The important thing is that you find your comfort level. Many people are fine with this workout level for the rest of their lives — it can boost your spirits and your health.

Want to take your program further? You've got the idea by now — simply add distance, go faster, or make the course harder (try hills). If you have to miss a workout, be sure to get back on track as soon as possible — good habits are hard to break!

It may take you three or four months to reach the goal of 3 miles five times a week — and that's fine. It's not a contest. You're doing this for yourself and your health. Your only opponent is inactivity.

Part V
The Part of Tens

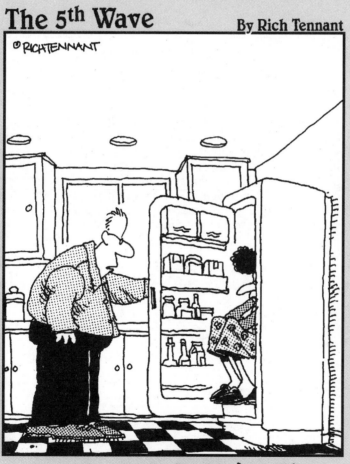

The 5th Wave   By Rich Tennant

"Having a hot flash, dear?"

In this part . . .

This just wouldn't be a *For Dummies* book without a yellow and black cover and a Part of Tens. We like to think of the Part of Tens as the icing on the cake — better yet, the fat-free whipped topping on the bowl of fruit. If you like top-ten lists, you've come to the right part of the book. In this part, we expose myths about menopause, give you the scoop on medical tests that you may run into, and outline some great ideas and programs that you can use to kick-start or jazz up your exercise routine.

Chapter 20

Menopause Myths Exposed

· ·

In This Chapter

▶ Ferreting out the realities of menopause

▶ Keeping sex sexy after the change

▶ Determining the accuracy of blood tests

· ·

*O*ne survey we recently came across shows that half of all women going through menopause feel unprepared and uninformed to face the change. Check out these common menopause myths and see how many of them you've heard — and how many you bought into! Because menopause and misconceptions go hand and hand so often, we couldn't limit ourselves to ten myths in this Part of Tens chapter.

You're Too Young to Be Menopausal in Your Thirties and Forties

Not really. Even though most women begin menopause sometime between 45 and 55 years of age (and the average age is 51), going through menopause earlier isn't impossible or unheard of. Making the situation seem even less cut and dry are those annoying symptoms, such as hot flashes, crying jags, mood swings, and interrupted sleep, that usually occur years before you actually quit having periods (official menopause). Those physical changes that characterize what most people refer to as the change are really more characteristic of *perimenopause* (the period of fluctuating hormone levels leading up to menopause). You can experience perimenopausal symptoms for a decade before the onset of menopause. So having hot flashes and fertility issues pop up when you're in your late thirties and early forties is perfectly normal.

But keep your gynecologist informed about your periods because skipping periods during your late thirties or early forties can also indicate medical problems. For some women, certain medical treatments cause the early onset of menopause, for example:

- Chemotherapy or radiation treatment may cause your ovaries to shut down early, depending on the type of treatments used.

- If you have both of your ovaries removed, you immediately experience *surgical menopause*. The ovaries, once responsible for producing the active form of estrogen that serves many bodily functions, are gone, and menopause begins.

- *Autoimmune disorders* (diseases of your immune system) and thyroid problems can result in *premature menopause* (menopause before age 40).

If you go through menopause earlier than most women, you may also increase your risk of developing menopause-related medical conditions, such as osteoporosis and cardiovascular disease, earlier. So talk to your doctor about ways you can prevent these conditions.

Menopause Is a Medical Condition that Must Be Treated

Not exactly. Remember puberty? Well menopause is puberty in reverse, with all the accompanying physical and emotional changes. (Sounds like a lot of fun when we put it that way, huh?) Menopause is not a medical condition in that it is not a disorder. It's a natural passage from your reproductive years to the rest of your life.

Menopause isn't a condition that requires medical attention any more than puberty requires medical attention. (The same degree of patience, however, is required.) The changes that take place are normal and natural. The care given to women on their journey through menopause is meant to alleviate discomfort and prevent disease rather than to interfere with the natural process. Many women don't experience any symptoms at all — they have no discomfort associated with the change, so there's nothing to treat. Other women find that herbs or a healthy lifestyle are effective in relieving symptoms. (We discuss the herbal route in Chapter 16, and Chapters 18 and 19 provide some great info on diet, nutrition, and exercise.) As it turns out, eating healthy and staying fit go a long way toward keeping your body and mind healthy without the estrogen they used to rely on.

Sometimes you need an extra biological boost, which can come in the forms of food supplements (calcium, for example) and hormone replacement therapy (HRT).

Because lower levels of estrogen over prolonged periods of time can result in other medical problems, work with your doctor to find appropriate therapies to prevent these problems.

Menopause Isn't a Disease, So There's No Need to See a Doctor

Think again. Menopause isn't a medical condition, but that fact doesn't mean you can ignore it. Your doctor must be aware of any new symptoms you experience or new medical issues that arise as you enter perimenopause and menopause.

Night sweats, fuzzy thinking, interrupted sleep, hot flashes, mood swings, fatigue, and irritability are recognized (and annoying) symptoms of perimenopause. But these symptoms can also signal more serious medical problems such as anemia, Epstein-Barr virus, thyroid problems, and other issues. You want to rule out the more serious medical issues before you assume that you're experiencing perimenopause symptoms. So keep track of your symptoms; write down when, how often, and for how long you experience them; and then share this information with your gynecologist or primary-care physician.

You may think that the main purpose of a visit to your doctor is to *assess* your current health and *fix* the related problems. But as you reach the point in your life at which most women enter perimenopause and menopause, your doctor will spend a greater amount of time trying to *prevent* the development of serious conditions including breast cancer, cervical cancer, hypertension, cardiovascular disease, high blood-cholesterol levels, and more.

You Lose the Urge to Have Sex after the Change

Hardly. Nearly half of menopausal women are satisfied with their sex life. If you do your own poll of your premenopausal friends (or tune into a daytime talk show), you'll probably find that the percentages are pretty comparable. Some women actually find sex more enjoyable — you don't have to worry about getting pregnant, you and your partner have some experience under your belts (so you know how to enjoy yourselves and your relationship), and you and your special someone may have more time to spend together.

That said, some women find intercourse to be painful because of vaginal dryness or vaginal atrophy. If vaginal dryness or atrophy is a problem for you, you can find some great remedies at the pharmacy or the grocery store. Vaginal moisturizers and vaginal estrogen pills or creams can be used regularly to treat vaginal dryness. Lubricants can be used during foreplay to eliminate painful intercourse.

Sexual stimulation begets sexual lubrication. In other words, the more you use it, the slower you lose it. Don't forget that "personal pleasure" can help you stay in shape. In fact, that famous sex doctor, Alfred Kinsey, found that even though marital intercourse declined as women got older, solitary sexual activity didn't decline until women were well past 60. Another study found that even though women's overall lubrication and sexual activity declined *slightly* after menopause, the frequency and pleasure of orgasm did not. For more about the change and your sex life (and making changes to your sex life), check out Chapter 8.

Irregular Vaginal Bleeding Always Means Cancer

Not exactly. Almost all perimenopausal women experience irregular menstrual cycles. In some months, you go 25 days between cycles; in others, you go 38 days. Some months are heavy, and others are light. Or you may even skip a month or two. These menstrual irregularities are generally caused by fluctuating hormones that get out of balance during perimenopause.

If you go through a super-absorbent pad or tampon every couple of hours, experience bleeding after intercourse, or experience bleeding more often than every three weeks, see your gynecologist to find out what's happening. Sometimes this type of irregular bleeding can signal more serious problems. Also, if you're bleeding between your menses, please consult your gynecologist.

Humps Accompany Old Age — End of Story

No way. Women don't automatically sprout a dowager's hump as they age. Vertebrae only collapse and result in spinal humps in some cases of *osteoporosis* (brittle bone disease).

If you don't want to acquire a hump, you need to begin strengthening your bones early in life by getting lots of calcium in your diet and exercise in your day. Osteoporosis is largely treatable with medicine and can often be prevented with the help of good nutrition, exercise, and calcium substitutes.

If your bones are in bad shape as you approach menopause, several drugs that can slow bone deterioration are on the market. The estrogen in hormone therapy also is very effective at slowing the rate of bone loss. A non-pharmaceutical approach to avoiding a hump is to add some regular strength-building exercises to your week.

Only HRT Can Relieve the Symptoms

False. Although hormone replacement therapy is a very effective way to eliminate many annoying menopausal symptoms, it's not the only way. But before we get to the matter at hand, we want to remind you that less than half of all women experience the symptoms we so often associate with menopause (or perimenopause). So you may get lucky and avoid these symptoms without any type of intervention. Also, remember that the symptoms, such as hot flashes, interrupted sleep, fuzzy thinking, mental lapses, and so on, are temporary and will eventually go away in their own time.

Now, if these symptoms are making your life miserable, you can try a number of different remedies. Start out by adopting a healthier lifestyle. Here are a few quick ideas (for more info, check out Chapters 18 and 19):

- ✔ Cut down on fats and junk foods.
- ✔ Eat only moderate amounts of meat and protein.
- ✔ Fill your plate with vegetables and fruits.
- ✔ Keep an eye on your alcohol intake. (Don't drink more than three to five alcoholic drinks a week.)
- ✔ Exercise at least three to five days a week for a half-hour each day.

You may also want to try an herbal remedy (such as black cohosh) or include some soy in your diet. Edamame (a type of large-seed soybean) and tofu are excellent sources of soy. (For more information on alternative ways to deal with the change, turn to Chapter 16.)

Women Don't Need to Worry about Heart Attacks

Wrong. Heart disease kills many more women each year than cancer does. In fact, the odds are that one out of two women will die of a heart attack or stroke. Estrogen seems to provide some protection to your cardiovascular system, so women generally have a lower risk of heart attack than men. After menopause, when you no longer produce estrogen, your risk of heart attack and stroke rises. A healthy diet and regular exercise can help lower your risk of cardiovascular disease.

Most Women Get Really Depressed During Menopause

False. Actually, women tend to get more depressed during the "procreation" years than during menopause. However, your emotions can take a tumble during perimenopause. Irritability, mood swings, and interrupted sleep can take a toll on your emotions. (For more information on the mental and emotional issues tied to menopause, peruse Chapter 9.) But you can find ways to alleviate these symptoms. A healthy diet and a regular exercise program help many women alleviate symptoms. Also a slew of pharmaceutical and herbal therapies can help resolve mental and emotional symptoms. (Take a look at Chapters 16 and 17.)

If you fought bouts of depression earlier in life, you may see a return of the symptoms during perimenopause, but remember that perimenopausal symptoms are transient and will go away in time. If you experience symptoms or signs of depression, talk to your doctor.

You'll Break a Bone if You Exercise Too Hard

Nope. Weight-bearing exercise (exercise that puts stress on your bones) is one of the best ways to help your body build bone. If you have osteoporosis or your bone density is getting low, the combination of weight-bearing exercise and calcium supplements (with vitamins D and K and magnesium) will prevent further bone loss.

If you've been living a sedentary lifestyle with little or no regular exercise (or you want to change your exercise regimen), discuss your exercise plan with a physician before you begin moving that body. Combining exercises that help your flexibility and balance with a walking program is a good way to get started. Flexibility and balance exercises can help you avoid falling and fractures. After you have that body moving, try adding some weight-bearing exercises to the routine. (Check out Chapter 19 for some terrific suggestions.)

A Blood Test Can Determine whether You're Going through Menopause

Well, here's the deal: Many gynecologists will test your levels of *follicle stimulating hormone* (FSH) to determine whether you're going through menopause. FSH is the hormone that tells the ovaries to get a follicle ready — this message kicks off your menstrual cycle. As your ovaries slow down, your brain tries to keep things moving at the regular pace, so it shoots out lots of FSH. Also, your brain doesn't see much estrogen coming back that says, "Alright already, the follicles are on their way," so FSH keeps on coming. Consistently high levels of FSH indicate the onset of menopause to the medical community.

But here's the catch: FSH levels will tell you when your ovaries are pretty close to shutting down follicle production, but they won't tell you if your hormones are in the wild state of fluctuation typical of the perimenopausal years. Unfortunately, most women are most interested in finding out what's going on with their bodies when they just start experiencing weird things like hot flashes, mood swings, and heart palpitations. By the time their FSH levels remain high, they've already figured the puzzle out — periods have pretty much stopped and the test just confirms the logical deduction that menopause is indeed near.

Chapter 21

More Than Ten Medical Tests for Menopausal Women

In This Chapter

▶ Uncovering common medical problems

▶ Making an annual trip to the gynecologist's office

▶ Relying on early detection of disease

*T*his chapter lists some basic health tests that help doctors identify diseases and other problems in their early stages — when they're more treatable. (We must confess that we include more than ten tests in this chapter, which kind of goes against the letter, but not the spirit, of the Part of Tens law.) *Early detection* is the key to successful treatment of nearly every disease that affects menopausal women. Avoiding the tests doesn't mean that you can avoid the related diseases, so visit your doctors regularly and follow through with their recommendations.

Pelvic Exam and Pap Smear

No one likes to put their feet in the stirrups and their privates in the saddle every year, but doing so sure helps you avoid some nasty problems down the line. You should have an annual gynecological exam. The gynecologist will check your female organs including your breasts, your vaginal tissue, your cervix, and your uterus. Your gynecologist will also perform a *Pap smear* to test for cervical cancer every year.

If you've had a complete hysterectomy for benign reasons, you should have a pelvic exam and Pap smear (to check for noncancerous medical issues) every year for three years, and then, the Pap can be done every three years. However, you still need a breast and pelvic exam every year.

Rectal Exam

Everyone squirms when this exam is the subject at hand. Everybody hates it, but the risks of postponing a rectal exam can be quite devastating to you and your loved ones. Regular rectal exams can help detect problems early — when they can be easily and painlessly treated. Part of this test is a *digital exam* in which the doctor checks your organs for signs of disease. The doctor inserts a gloved finger into your rectum to evaluate the health of your tissues. Keep in mind that the long-term benefits greatly outweigh the short-term unpleasantness of the procedure. And also remember that your doctor *chose* this field of medicine.

The other part of this exam is a *fecal occult test,* which enables doctors to check whether you have blood in your stool. This part of the test is necessary because the presence of blood can be an indication of problems, such as cancer, in your colon.

You should have a rectal exam once a year during your annual gynecological physical, especially after age 50.

Colonoscopy

Colon cancer is a form of cancer that progresses very slowly and is readily treatable. But it's the third leading cause of cancer deaths among American women. No one likes the test — it's that simple. And women avoid discussing the issue until they have symptoms. The problem is that patients very often don't experience any symptoms until the disease is in an advanced stage — a point when successful treatment is much more difficult.

While performing a colonoscopy, your doctor can find and remove precancerous polyps (doctors know them as *adenomatous polyps*) before they have a chance of becoming cancerous. The night before your colonoscopy, you drink a potion that helps clean out your colon. While you're under the influence of a light sedative, the doctor inserts a flexible scope into your colon that allows her to view the colon walls in search of polyps or other unhealthy tissue. If she finds a polyp, she can remove it and send it to the lab for analysis. Lab analysis determines if the polyp is benign or precancerous.

Want to cut your risk of colon cancer by one-third? All you have to do is regularly schedule (and go through with) a colonoscopy. If you're over 50, have a colonoscopy every five years — more often if you have polyps.

Bone-Density Screening

It's really best to have at least one bone-density screening before you're menopausal. When you're 40, visit your doctor and get a baseline bone-density screening. The results provide your doctors with something to compare future screenings to. If you show signs of bone loss in this or subsequent tests, you'll have bone screenings every two years.

If your family has a history of osteoporosis (your sister, mother, or grand-mother have osteoporosis), get a baseline bone-density screening when you're in your late thirties.

If you've never had a bone screening and you're over 40, talk to your doctor about your options.

Mammogram

Early detection is the key to reducing your risk of breast cancer, so you should begin getting annual mammograms when you're 40 years old with a baseline taken at age 35. If your mother or sister has had breast cancer, get your first mammogram even earlier, when you're 30.

The American Cancer Society recommends that you get a mammogram every one to two years after age 40 and every year after you turn 50. Other groups advise less frequent mammograms. In our opinion, annual mammograms are your best bet even if scientists are still debating the merits of a yearly regimen.

Cholesterol Screening

A cholesterol screening checks your total cholesterol, *LDL cholesterol* (bad cholesterol), *HDL cholesterol* (good cholesterol), and *triglycerides* (another form of fat found in your blood) and computes your cholesterol ratio. Take this simple blood test every five years. You should take it when you're fasting — nothing to eat or drink for 12 hours before the test. If your doctor identifies problems with your cholesterol or triglyceride levels or you have a history of high blood pressure, diabetes, thyroid problems, or obesity, your doctor may want to screen you more frequently.

Fasting Blood-Glucose Test

Adult-onset diabetes can lead to coronary heart disease, so you want to diagnose this problem early. Begin having your blood sugar (*glucose*) tested when you're 20 and repeat the test every three to five years — more frequently if you experience problems. The blood-glucose test is a simple blood test administered after you've had nothing to eat or drink for 12 hours (that's where the *fasting* part of the name comes from). You can also screen for diabetes by checking for sugar in your urine.

Thyroid Screening

The symptoms of thyroid problems and the symptoms of menopause can be quite similar. Get your first thyroid screening at age 35. The screening measures your levels of thyroid-stimulating hormone (THS) and thyroid antibodies.

CA 125 Test

Doctors don't routinely perform this blood test during your annual gynecological exam. But you may want to take it if you have a family history of ovarian cancer or if you're having abdominal bloating or pain or other symptoms that evade diagnosis or don't respond to other treatments. Levels of the CA 125 antigen often rise with the presence of ovarian cancer, endometriosis, ovarian cysts, fibroids, and even the early stages of pregnancy.

This exam isn't considered a diagnostic test for ovarian cancer because higher levels of CA 125 don't necessarily indicate ovarian cancer, and sometimes, levels don't rise if you have ovarian cancer. But high levels of CA 125 can be an early warning of ovarian cancer and cause your doctor to pursue additional tests until ovarian cancer can be ruled out.

Ovarian Hormone Screening

Out of necessity, the standard practice for prescribing hormone therapy is a method of trial and error — a "try this regimen and let me know how you feel" kind of approach. Everybody processes hormones differently, so the amount of hormone in a medication isn't the amount that reaches your bloodstream.

For example, the same form of estrogen may affect two women differently. And your body may respond better to some estrogens than others.

The key to what "works" and what doesn't is the amount of *estradiol* (the active form of estrogen) your body produces in response to the estrogen you're taking. The only accurate way to know how much estradiol you're churning out is to draw blood and analyze it for hormone levels. (Saliva tests are available, but they're less accurate.)

That said, the majority of doctors stick with the standard dosing formulas and do the trial-and-error thing until you tell them you're feeling better. We just want you to know that an alternative (ovarian hormone screening) is available and a bit more objective. Estradiol levels below 90 pg/ml result in the typical hot flashes, interrupted sleep, mood swings, and other annoying perimenopausal symptoms. If your levels drop below 80 or 90 pg/ml, you risk suffering from bone loss and cardiovascular issues. So the key is to get your estradiol levels up to 90 or 100 pg/ml after menopause.

Sometime during your twenties or thirties, you should have a hormone screening to check your premenopausal baseline levels of estrogen, progesterone, and testosterone at two points in your menstrual cycle — Day 1 or 2 of your cycle and then again at around Day 18 (assuming a 28-day cycle). The technician draws some blood and sends it to a lab for analysis. The results give you an idea of your typical hormone levels prior to menopause.

But never having had a baseline drawn is okay — you can still benefit from ovarian hormone screening. If you've been experimenting with hormone therapy and want to get off the roller coaster, you may want to ask your doctor to check out your current hormone levels to see how effectively your therapy is working.

Stress Test

You may think that your life has been one big stress test, but actually, a stress test is a legitimate medical procedure. A stress test is basically an electro-cardiogram (EKG) that a technician performs while you walk on a treadmill. You may have had an EKG in the past to qualify for life insurance or as part of an annual exam. The purpose of the test is to see how your heart responds to the stress of exercise. If you're overweight, have high blood pressure, or experience chest pain or shortness of breath with mild exertion, your doctor may suggest a stress test. Your doctor may also perform a stress test to check out your heart before you begin a new exercise program.

The procedure is simple. A technician sticks some electrical wires on your chest to record the electrical activity in your heart. This information tells the doctor if your heart is getting enough oxygen or if it's been damaged. To stress your heart, you walk on a special treadmill while you're plugged into the EKG.

You should take a stress test if your doctor suspects that you have coronary artery disease; otherwise, get a baseline reading at 40 and then take the test every three to five years. The risk of heart attack rises after menopause, so don't overlook the importance of checking out the health of your heart.

Chapter 22

Ten Terrific Fitness Programs For Menopausal Women

- -

In This Chapter

▶ Walking your way to better health

▶ Swimming for shore

▶ Developing a hankering for yoga

- -

*N*eed help getting your fitness program off the ground? In this chapter, we provide some great suggestions to help you clear the runway.

Many women dread the thought of a workout, because to them, the concept implies sweat, finding time that they don't have, and too much effort. If this description fits you, think again. You can find a workout that fits your schedule and your desired level of energy output. (If you hate to sweat, check out the water-based workouts we include in this chapter.)

Be sure to warm up and cool down for five to ten minutes before and after you workout. If you have trouble with your heart, blood pressure, cholesterol, or diabetes, if you suffer from a respiratory condition, if you're overweight, if you smoke, or if you've been a couch potato for more years than you can remember, discuss your physical-fitness plans with your doctor before getting started. And think of your weekly fitness routine as a buffet. Include a little of everything on your plate — aerobic training, strength training, and flexibility and balance-building exercises.

Core-Stability Training

Core-stability training is a great way to improve your balance and flexibility, reduce your risk of injury, and lessen your amount of soreness associated with performing daily activities. Core stability training is basically strength training that targets the muscle groups that make up the core of your body — the abdominal, lower-back, hip, and pelvic muscles are the primary focus. Strengthening your core muscles allows them to do their job (maintaining your body's stability and balance) better.

These muscles are the foundation of support for just about any activity your body does. The everyday aches and pains that many woman feel are often the result of weakened core-muscle groups. Your body tries to compensate for these weak muscles, which can lead to pain in your lower back and arm and leg joints.

Here's how core-stability training works: You incorporate exercises that challenge your abdominal, lower-back, hip, pelvic, and oblique muscles. You can strengthen these muscles with traditional exercises and callisthenic-type movements. (Chapter 19 is full of great exercises to help you strengthen these muscles, and we include even more resources in Appendix B.)

Some additional toys are available that can add variety and fun to your workout and make your workout more effective. Equipment such as balance balls, stability boards, and old-fashioned medicine balls makes targeting the muscles that help maintain your stability and balance easier. Strengthening these muscles can also improve your posture.

Walking

Walking is an inexpensive and convenient way to relieve stress, improve your fitness, and build muscle tone. However, only 6 percent of people who get all their exercise from walking meet the U.S. Surgeon General's guidelines for fitness. To make sure that your efforts bring you good health, walk

- For at least 30 minutes per session.
- At least four times a week.
- At a moderately intense pace. You should cover about 3½ miles in an hour (or 1¾ miles in a half an hour).

Chapter 19 has a whole section on how to design a walking program.

Elliptical Training

The elliptical-training machine is a relatively new but terrific way to get aerobic exercise without hurting your joints with high-impact workouts. An elliptical trainer looks like a combination of a treadmill and a climber that grew arms! The machine is called an elliptical trainer because your feet move in the shape of an oval during the workout instead of back and forth like they do on a treadmill or up and down like they move on a climber. Because your feet follow an oval path, the exercise is low impact but still provides a full range of motion for your legs. The arms on the machine go back and forth while you stride, so you get a total body workout.

Running

Running reduces your risk for developing heart disease, high blood pressure, adult-onset diabetes, and several types of cancer. It also increases the levels of good (HDL) cholesterol in your blood, which helps you get rid of the bad (LDL) cholesterol. (For more information on cholesterol levels, see Chapter 5.) Running also improves your cardiovascular and respiratory systems and can help you control your weight. (Some people lose up to 12 pounds the first year they start running without reducing the calories they eat.)

Getting started on a running regimen is easy; all you need to do is chart out a course (in a safe area) and get a pair of good running shoes. If you're a beginner, try running a mile. If you can't do a mile, try alternating between running and walking until you can cover the entire mile without the walking part. Then add a little distance at a time. Initially schedule about 30 minutes of running time and build up the duration as you go.

Swimming

Swimming is easy on your joints and helps build muscle strength equally on both sides of your body. In fact, swimming forces you to use all of your muscles. Now that's what we call a workout! It's a great exercise for people looking to increase their overall physical fitness or recover from an injury.

If you've had a hip or knee replaced or you suffer from arthritis, swimming is an excellent way to maintain aerobic conditioning through low-impact exercise.

Cycling

Perhaps walking and running are too slow for you, and you're not really a water person. Taking up cycling, whether in the gym or on the road, may be for you. Cycling is a great aerobic workout that improves your cardiovascular health, muscle tone, and stamina.

If you're just getting started, you may want to try a stationary bike at your local YMCA or health club. Try riding for six minutes at 15 miles per hour (or 55 revolutions per minute), five times a week. Gradually work up to 20 to 25 minutes, five times a week, at the same speed. As you become accustomed to cycling, you can build your aerobic fitness even more by increasing your speed.

After spending some time in the saddle, you may want to try a spin class. A *spin class* is a group indoor-cycling class that can really help you build your aerobic fitness. You can find spin classes at many YMCA locations, community colleges, and health clubs across the country. An instructor guides each class and makes your "ride" on a special stationary bike as challenging as you like.

If you're more of the outdoor type, get that bicycle out of the garage, check the brakes and tires, and take it out for a ride. Don't forget about safety: Always wear a helmet and choose a course in a safe neighborhood that has little traffic and contains few hills.

Start by riding for ten minutes on a relatively flat course (preferably away from traffic) five times a week. Add two minutes to your workout each week (riding five times a week) so that by the end of Week 11 you're riding for 30 minutes five times a week.

Yoga

Yoga is a great way to improve your health. Studies have shown that yoga can reduce stress, lower blood pressure, relieve arthritis, and build strength and flexibility. The breathing techniques used during a yoga workout help increase the oxygen levels in your blood.

Some styles of yoga focus more on spiritual aspects, such as meditation or chanting, and are great for stress reduction and relaxation. Other forms focus on body alignment and challenging workouts that improve muscle tone, balance, and flexibility. All forms of yoga use poses and breathing techniques to heighten the mind-body connection. You can pull out your copy of *Yoga For Dummies* (Georg Feuerstein, Wiley Publishing, Inc.) for more information. What? Don't have one? You may want to check it out.

T'ai Chi

T'ai chi helps stretch and tone muscles, relieve stress, and improve balance and circulation. You may even lower your blood pressure. This ancient, Chinese form of exercise, meditation, and self-defense involves controlled movements done slowly and continuously. The forms are similar to those used in other martial arts. If T'ai Chi sounds like it may be up your alley, *T'ai Chi For Dummies* (Therese Iknoian with Manny Fuentes, Wiley Publishing, Inc.) is one place to start.

Pilates

Even though Pilates (puh-*lah*-teez) entered fitness centers fairly recently, its roots actually date back to the 1920s. You can think of Pilates as a combination of yoga, stretching, and calisthenics all rolled up into one set of exercises.

These exercises work on many of the same muscle groups as a core-stability-training program (check out our "Core-Stability Training" section earlier in this chapter) and offer many of the same advantages. In Pilates, you perform slow, extremely focused movements that work the muscles in your abdomen, lower back, and buttocks. And yes, there's a snazzy yellow-and-black covered book on this subject too — *Pilates For Dummies* (Ellie Herman, Wiley Publishing, Inc.).

Water Aerobics

Here's a great exercise for women who feel out of place jumping around in an aerobics class in front of a bunch of other people. Why's it so great? Your legs are under water — if you miss a step or have to take a breather, no one's the wiser. Water aerobics helps you work your cardiovascular system, arm muscles, and leg muscles. It's less stressful on your joints than a lot of exercise programs, and it improves your balance and coordination. Many health clubs and YMCA locations offer classes led by professional trainers. Water aerobics is a great way to have fun, stay cool, and get active.

Part VI
Appendixes

The 5th Wave   By Rich Tennant

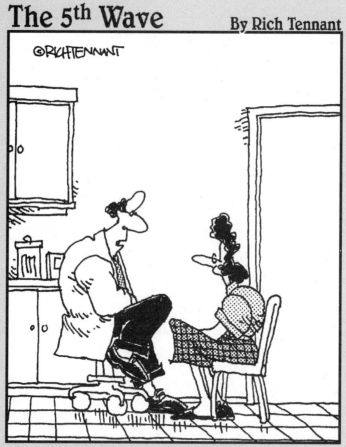

"Sudden perspiration, shallow breathing, and rapid heart rate are all signs of menopause. The fact that those symptoms only occur when the pool boy is working in your backyard, however, raises some questions."

In this part . . .

Literature on menopause is often filled with a dazzling array of medical terms, jargon, and other overstuffed phrases. We, of course, try to simplify this state of affairs. But, in case you run across a word that you need a quick definition for, whether it's in this book or other literature about menopause, we include a glossary of terms — Appendix A. In Appendix B, we provide you with a bunch of additional sources of information — from books to Web sites — that do a great job covering menopause and other health-related issues of interest to women.

Appendix A

Glossary

· ·

Adenomatous polyp: Pre-cancerous *polyp* in the lining of the colon.

Amenorrhea: Condition in women who haven't gone through *menopause* in which they miss menstrual periods for several months in a row.

Androgens: Hormones that produce masculine effects on the body such as a deep voice and facial hair. Both men and women produce androgens, although women produce them in much smaller amounts.

Angina: Pain in the chest, arm, or neck caused by lack of blood flow to the heart. Angina is often a symptom of *coronary artery disease.*

Antioxidant: A substance, such as vitamins A, C, E, or beta-carotene, that protects cells from damaging *oxidation,* which appears to encourage aging and certain diseases.

Arteriosclerosis: See *atherosclerosis.*

Atherosclerosis: *Cholesterol* and other substances building up in the walls of blood vessels. This process causes a narrowing of the blood vessels. People used to refer to this condition as *hardening of the arteries.* It can lead to *coronary artery disease.*

Atrophy: See *vaginal atrophy.*

Bisphosphonates: A group of medications used to treat *osteoporosis* that stimulate bone growth and slow down bone destruction.

Body Mass Index (BMI): A method of estimating body fat using a weight-to-height ratio. For weight in pounds and height in inches, BMI = Weight/Height^2 × 704.5.

Carcinoma *in situ:* Condition in which abnormal cancer cells are located in a confined space and haven't spread to other areas. At this stage, most cancers can be successfully treated.

Cardiovascular disease (CVD): Disease that affects the heart, arteries, veins, and capillaries.

Cholesterol: A fat-like substance that comprises an important part of the body's cells. Three forms of cholesterol are found in blood: high-density lipids **(HDL),** low-density lipids **(LDL),** and very-low-density lipids (VLDL). Found in all foods made from animals.

Combination therapy: A type of hormone therapy in which a woman takes an *estrogen* and a *progestogen.*

Conjugated estrogens: A mixture of estrogens sometimes used in *hormone therapy.* They're chemically different from human *estrogen* and can come from either plants or horses.

Continuous combination therapy: A type of hormone therapy regimen in which a woman takes an *estrogen* and *progestogen* together throughout the month.

Coronary artery disease (CAD): A disease in which the blood vessels that feed the heart become narrow and restrict blood flow to the heart. *Atherosclerosis* is the process that leads to coronary artery disease.

Coronary heart disease (CHD): Damage to the heart resulting from *coronary artery disease.* Because the terms are so similar, many people use them interchangeably.

Corpus luteum: A yellow sac formed from the remains of the *follicle* after the follicle releases the egg. The corpus luteum produces *progesterone.*

Cyclic combination therapy: A type of hormone therapy regimen in which a woman takes estrogen by itself for several days of the month, followed by a period in which she takes *estrogen* and *progestogen.*

Deep vein thrombosis (DVT): Blood clots in the veins near the bones that are surrounded by muscle (usually the upper arm, thigh, or pelvic areas). These veins lie deeper under the skin than surface veins and return more blood to the heart. A clot in one of these veins often causes more complications than a clot in surface veins causes.

DEXA: Abbreviation for *dual-energy x-ray absorptiometry* — a method of measuring bone-mineral density. Used to screen for *osteoporosis.*

DHEA: Abbreviation for *dehydroepiandrosterone,* which is a male hormone produced in a woman's adrenal glands and *ovaries.*

Dowager's hump: An old slang term for an apparent hump in the back of some people with osteoporosis. Caused by the collapse of vertebrae in the spine due to porous (brittle) bone. The term comes from the outdated idea that osteoporosis is a condition that only strikes postmenopausal women (little old ladies, or dowagers).

Endometrium: The lining of the uterus.

Estradiol: The active form of *estrogen* made in the *ovaries* prior to *menopause.* The most potent form of estrogen in humans. Plays a role in many bodily functions.

Estriol: Form of *estrogen* only produced during pregnancy.

Estrogen: A female hormone produced in the *ovaries* and in the adrenal glands.

Estrogen receptor: A "docking station" on a cell that allows that particular body part to make use of *estrogen.* Estrogen receptors are located all over a woman's body but are highly concentrated in estrogen-sensitive tissues such as uterus and breast tissue.

Estrone: A type of *estrogen* made by the *ovaries,* adrenal glands, and body fat before *menopause.* After menopause, body fat makes estrone; therefore, estrone is the only type of estrogen in good supply after menopause. Estrone is less active than *estradiol* estrogen.

Fibrinogen: A type of protein that helps blood clot.

Follicle: A little sac created from an *oocyte* (seed) in the ovary. The follicle produces estrogen in the ovary. At least one of these little guys releases an egg each month during a woman's reproductive years. After the egg is released, the follicle is called a *corpus luteum.*

Follicle-stimulating hormone (FSH): A hormone produced in the brain that triggers the *ovaries* to begin developing *follicles.* Doctors consider continued high levels of FSH to be an indication of *menopause.* The FSH keeps trying to stimulate follicle production when the cupboard is bare — the ovary can no longer crank out follicles — which is a sign that the ovary is entering retirement and you're entering menopause.

HDL: Abbreviation for high-density lipid. HDL is "good" cholesterol because it can carry fat from the body cells back to the liver for excretion. *Lipids* are made up of protein and fat. Lipids with more protein than fat are called high-density lipids; a lipid with more fat than protein is called a low-density lipid *(LDL).*

Hormone: Chemicals produced in organs that travel through the body to activate functions in other parts of the body.

Hormone-receptor site: A "docking station" for hormones on a cell where hormones can connect to cells to manipulate them.

Hormone replacement therapy (HRT): See *hormone therapy.*

Hormone therapy (HT): Treatment designed to adjust hormone levels using synthetic or natural female hormones. Doctors generally administer this treatment to women going through *perimenopause* and/or *menopause.*

Hypertension: Another name for high blood pressure.

Hysterectomy: Surgical removal of the uterus. A *simple hysterectomy* removes only the uterus. A *complete hysterectomy* removes the uterus and the *ovaries.* A complete hysterectomy causes *surgical menopause.*

Incontinence: The inability to "hold it" or keep from urinating.

Interstitial cystitis (IC): A bladder condition that's hard to diagnose, but the symptoms include mild discomfort, pressure, tenderness, or intense pain in the bladder and surrounding pelvic area. Symptoms may include an urgent need to urinate (*urgency*), a frequent need to urinate (*frequency*), or a combination of these symptoms. Researchers don't know the causes of IC, and few treatments are effective.

Isoflavone: See *phytoestrogen.*

Labia: The lips of the vaginal opening. **See also *vulva.***

LDL: Abbreviation for low-density lipid. LDLs are found in the bloodstream and are thought to carry cholesterol from the liver to body cells. Eating a diet high in saturated fats and cholesterol will raise your LDL levels. The higher the LDL level, the greater the incidence of heart attack or *coronary artery disease.*

Libido: Sex drive.

Lobules: Milk-producing glands in the breast. Cancer sometimes starts in the lobules.

Luteinizing hormone (LH): A hormone made in the pituitary gland. In women, it triggers *ovulation.*

Menarche: The onset of menstrual periods, which signals the beginning of a woman's reproductive maturation.

Menopause: The technical meaning is the end of menstruation — no *menses* for 12 months. Because periods are so irregular in the months leading up to menopause, the medical community generally doesn't consider you to be officially menopausal until 12 months after your last period. The media uses this term pretty loosely by using it to refer to all stages of menopause including *perimenopause,* menopause, and *postmenopause.* In this book, we restrict usage of the term to the stage after a woman is officially menopausal.

Menses: This word is derived from the Latin word for *month.* The term refers to your period — the periodic flow of blood from the uterus.

Osteoblast: Cells that build new bone.

Osteoclast: Cells that break down bone during the bone-maintenance process.

Osteopenia: Loss of bone density that isn't sufficiently severe to be called *osteoporosis.* If action isn't taken to better maintain the bone, this condition will turn into osteoporosis over time.

Osteoporosis: Loss of bone density. Makes bones brittle, porous, and weak.

Ovaries: Female sex organs that store "seeds" (*oocytes*), some of which develop into *follicles.* You're born with two ovaries. They produce the hormones *estrogen* and *progesterone* as well as a small amount of *testosterone.*

Ovulation: The process by which the egg is released from the *follicle.*

Oxidation: Technically, this term refers to the process through which oxygen combines with another substance — like when metal turns to rust. So what does this have to do with menopause? Unstable oxygen molecules, *free radicals* in med speak, are produced as your body's cells go about their daily chores. Because they're unstable, free radicals react with other molecules as they move through your body. Oxidation does some good things, but it also damages healthy cells, which can lead to cancer, heart disease, and other ailments common to menopausal women.

Palpitation: In this book, we use the term to refer to a rapid heartbeat.

Perimenopause: Time frame prior to *menopause* when hormones fluctuate radically, periods may be irregular, and women may experience physical and emotional symptoms (such as hot flashes, heart palpitations, mood swings, irritability, and crying jags). Perimenopause may begin ten years prior to menopause but more typically begins four to six years prior to menopause and continues through the first year after menstrual periods stop.

Phytoestrogen: *Estrogen* produced by plants (such as the soybean plant) that binds with human *estrogen receptors* and results in estrogen-like actions. Sometimes called *isoflavone.*

Polyp: A noncancerous growth that protrudes from tissues. In this book, we discuss colon polyps.

Postmenopause: The years after *menopause* when the ovaries have stopped functioning. This is the time when health conditions associated with long periods of low *estrogen* (*osteoporosis* and *cardiovascular disease*) are your top concern.

Premature menopause: Experiencing menopause at an unusually early age (like in your thirties). Premature menopause leaves you at risk of osteoporosis and higher cholesterol fairly early in life.

Premenopausal: Term associated with women who haven't yet gone through *menopause.*

Progesterone: A female hormone produced by the *ovaries* after *ovulation* to prepare the uterus for fertilization.

Progestin: Synthetic form of the natural hormone *progesterone.*

Progestogen: Any hormone, natural or synthetic, that has the same effect on the body as *progesterone.*

Pulmonary embolism: Blockage of an artery in the lungs by a blood clot.

Sequential combination therapy: A type of hormone therapy regimen in which a woman takes estrogen, followed by progestogen, followed by a period in which no hormones are taken.

SERMs: Abbreviation for *selective estrogen receptor modulators* — special "designer hormones" used in *hormone therapy.* They can activate *estrogen receptors* in some parts of the body while blocking estrogen receptors in other parts of the body. SERMs are particularly useful for women who want the benefits of HT but don't want to increase their risk for breast cancer.

Serotonin: A brain chemical that regulates sleep, mood, *libido,* pain, and more.

Surgical menopause: *Menopause* that is the result of the surgical removal of the ovaries.

Testosterone: A male hormone produced by the *ovaries* in low levels. Helps maintain muscle mass, bone, and *libido* in women.

Transdermal: A method of delivering medication in which the medication is absorbed through the skin and goes directly into the bloodstream.

Triglyceride: A chemical form of the fats that circulate in the bloodstream and are used by the body to make *cholesterol.*

Unopposed estrogen: A type of hormone therapy regimen in which a woman uses *estrogen* without *progestogen* to balance it.

Urethra: The little canal through which you urinate.

Urinary-tract infection (UTI): An infection that affects the bladder, *urethra,* or kidneys.

Vaginal atrophy: Thinning and drying of vaginal tissue often experienced during *perimenopause* and *menopause.*

Vulva: Collective term for the external genital organs that are visible between a woman's thighs consisting of the *mons* (fleshy, rounded area covered by pubic hair), *labia* (lips or folds of the vagina), *hymen* (thin mucous membrane that keeps the vagina partially closed), *clitoris* (a woman's pleasure spot), and some glands.

Appendix B

Resources

● ●

*I*f you're interested in finding more information about menopause, hormones, and related conditions, here's a quick guide to some terrific resources.

Fabulous Books about Menopause, Health, Fitness, and Related Issues

These are some of our favorite reference books. They contain some good information, and the authors wrote them with the layperson in mind. You can find these books at your local library or bookstore.

The Aerobics Program for Total Well Being: Exercise/Diet/Emotional Balance, by Kenneth H. Cooper (Bantam Doubleday Dell, 1997). Okay, this book was first introduced in 1985, but it still works. If you only get one book about maintaining your well-being, get this one. Whether you're just getting started or you have 20 marathons under your belt, you'll take something away from reading this book. Exercise, diet, and emotional balance are key to keeping your cardiovascular system and bones healthy — just the parts that trouble menopausal women.

The Cooper Clinic Solution to the Diet Revolution, by Georgia G. Kostas (Balancing Act Nutrition Books, 2001). This book is a fabulous source for getting healthy and staying that way. You can find out how to eat right to lose weight or maintain your current healthy weight. Kostas packs a bunch of great advice on foods and exercise between these two covers. Order directly from Cooper Clinic by calling 972-560-2655.

Dr. Susan Love's Hormone Book, by Susan Love and Karen Lindsey (Random House, 1997). This book is a bit dated, given all the new studies that have been released recently, but most of Love's conclusions still hold up. It presents a very balanced approach to menopause and hormone therapy.

Getting Stronger: Weight Training for Men and Women (Revised Edition), by Bill Pearl (Shelter Publications, 2001). Many women really don't know where to start when they're first told to incorporate weight-bearing exercise into their workout. If you're a bit perplexed about the subject, pick up this title. You can find out what to look for in a health club, how to use different types of weight machines, how to condition specific muscles, and how to create a workout program to get in shape for your favorite sport. Nice illustrations accompany all exercise descriptions and show you exactly what to do and what muscle you'll work.

Healthy Women, Healthy Lives, by Susan E. Hankinson, Graham A. Colditz, JoAnn E. Manson, and Frank E. Speizer (Simon & Schuster, 2001). With that many authors, it has to be good. *Healthy Women, Healthy Lives* offers important lessons about reducing your risk for many chronic diseases and several forms of cancer. Using results from one of the largest studies of women in the world, the Nurses' Health Study, this resource can help you make better-informed personal-health choices. It's informative, yet very easy to read and understand.

Muscle Mechanics, by Everett Aagberg (Human Kinetics Publishers, 1998). If fantastic illustrations for tons of exercises that cover every major muscle group in your body sounds like something you can use, Aagberg has a book for you. This is a great book for women who want to take the next step in their exercise program — whether you want to improve your muscle tone or simply get into better shape. You can even get help designing a customized exercise program just for you.

Screaming to be Heard: Hormone Connections Women Suspect and Doctors Still Ignore, by Elizabeth Lee Vliet (M. Evans and Company, 2001). This book is a terrific resource if you want to know how your natural hormones work and how menopause changes things. The title reflects the author's indignation at the lack of solid research and medical training in the field of hormone therapy. Vliet draws upon her medical experience and uses scenarios and cases from her professional encounters.

Stretching, by Bob Anderson (Shelter Publications, 2000). This book is celebrating its 20th anniversary, and it's still the bible on the subject of stretching. The updates include new stretches for inline skating and rock climbing (not too popular 20 years ago), but the title stays faithful to its original principle that people of all ages and abilities need to stay flexible and fit to keep well. If you're currently a couch potato, start with this book. It contains stretches that take you from square one and prepare you for an exercise program. For the more-active woman, *Stretching* offers treasures that can help you push your sport or exercise performance to the next level.

Strong Women Stay Young, by Miriam E. Nelson with Sarah Wernick (Bantam Doubleday Dell, 1998). Go for it girl. Here's the book you need to learn how aerobic exercise and strength training build and maintain healthy bone and muscle.

Woman's Body: A Manual For Life, by Miriam Stoppard (DK Publishing, 1995). This book covers menopause and a whole range of other mental and physical issues you may face throughout your lifetime.

Wonderful Web Sites for Women

If you have access to the Internet, the world of health and nutrition is literally at your fingertips. In this section, we list some of our favorite Web sites. These sites have our personal seal of approval because they have tons of up-to-date information and provide links to lots of other Web sites.

American Herbalist Guild

www.americanherbalistsguild.com

If you're interested in finding an herbalist in the United States, check out this site. It gives you the organization's code of ethics as well as links to the Web sites of its members. Those of you interested in learning more about herbs will also enjoy the educational programs listed and online courses provided on this page.

American Medical Women's Association

www.amwa-doc.org

You can find information about many women's medical issues on this site. It's geared toward women physicians, but the lay person can read the latest about many health topics, particularly hormone therapy, osteoporosis, and other conditions important to menopausal women.

American Yoga Association

www.americanyogaassociation.org

Find an instructor, take a free class, or learn more about the history of yoga. This site is a great place to visit for people just getting interested in yoga and for yoga vets who want more info.

Dietary Guidelines for Americans 2000

www.health.gov/dietaryguidelines/dga2000/document/frontcover.htm

Here's a Web site that gives you the latest on diet and fitness recommendations from the U.S. Department of Health and Human Services. It's quick and gets right to the point.

FitDay.com

www.fitday.com

This site bills itself as "Your online diet and fitness journal," and it's the handiest little site on the Internet if you're trying to eat healthier or lose weight. It lets you type in the foods you eat, and it tells you the calories and nutrients found in each. You can also keep track of your food consumption after every meal (or even plan your calories ahead of time). Because the site also keeps track of nutrients, you can make sure your diet is balanced. For women trying to lose weight, FitDay.com has some nice planners and exercise trackers so you can see if you're going to lose weight with your current eating and exercise routines. And the best part? It's all free!

National Center for Complementary and Alternative Medicine Clearinghouse

www.nccam.nih.gov

This site provides information on alternative medical therapies not commonly used or previously accepted in conventional Western medicine. We particularly like the "Health Information" page because it has links to alerts and advisories that warn you of any harmful therapies on the market. You can also search for information on the particular therapy or condition that interests you.

National Osteoporosis Foundation

www.nof.org

You can find lots of information on osteoporosis on this Web site. Because osteoporosis is such a big concern for women after menopause, you may want to refer to this page often. The site features news about osteoporosis, prevention, and treatment, a find-a-doctor feature, and the opportunity to sign up for a weekly newsletter.

National Women's Health Information Center

www.4woman.gov/faq/hormone.htm

This site is provided by the U.S. Department of Health and Human Services. The Web address listed above leads to an area that offers details on the Women's Health Initiative study concerning the risks and benefits of one type of hormone therapy — combination therapy of conjugated equine estrogen and MPA progestin. The information is nicely organized, and you can get right to the issues that concern you. Links to a variety of government and medical groups of interest to women after menopause are also included. By clicking on "Home" link, you can visit the center's homepage, which contains information on a wide variety of health issues related to women.

North American Menopause Society

www.menopause.org

This Web site is dedicated to promoting women's health during midlife and beyond through an understanding of menopause. It contains tons of information on perimenopause, early menopause, menopausal symptoms, long-term health effects of estrogen loss, and a wide variety of therapies to enhance your health.

Ontario Herbalists Association

www.herbalists.on.ca

Looking for an herbalist in or around Ontario? Here's a great Web site that publishes its code of ethics and provides a listing of member herbalists by location. The site is also a treasure trove of educational material and seminars for those of you who want to learn more about the practice.

WebMD

www.webmd.com

Now here's a terrific site to find out about what ails you (or what you think might ail you). It has a powerful search engine. You can type in the name of a medical condition or medication and get a list of articles that may be helpful to you. Nearly all the information is user friendly and written for the average person who isn't a medical expert. All the articles are kept current and accurate.

Women and Cardiovascular Disease

www.women.americanheart.org

Don't let the name scare you. The information here can help you *prevent* cardiovascular disease. This Web address takes you to the part of the American Heart Association's site devoted to women. You can find information on women's risks of heart disease, cardiovascular problems, and stroke. This site is full of up-to-the-minute, heart-healthy information and includes links to other cardiovascular-related Web sites.

Women's Cancer Network

www.wcn.org

The Women's Cancer Network, which can answer many of your questions about gynecologic cancer, is hosted by the Society of Gynecologic Oncologists. You can find everything from the most recent research results to physician referrals here.

Women's Health Initiative

www.nhlbi.nih.gov/whi/whi.htm

The Women's Health Initiative is a huge research project (sponsored by the National Institutes of Health) that studies — what else? — women's health. To be more specific, this project is a 15-year, on-going study focusing on post-menopausal women. The Women's Health Initiative has made major contributions to our understanding of menopause and hormone therapy. The study is scheduled to be completed in 2005, but results are already coming in. This site gives you some background on the study.

www.whi.org

Consider this listing a two-for-one bonus. This site is actually supposed to be for participants in the Women's Health Initiative study, but it has some terrific information on the study's results that have already been published. Also, the section concerning HRT in the news is great because it provides links to all the media coverage of the study's already-published results concerning hormone therapy.

Index

• *F* •

• I •

• J •

• K •

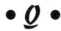

NOW AVAILABLE!

FOR DUMMIES Videos & DVDs

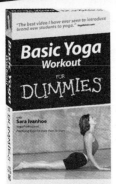
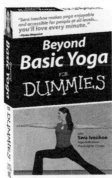
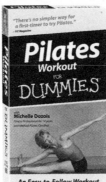
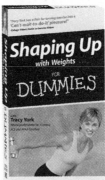
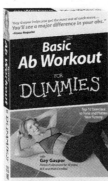
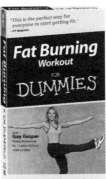
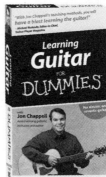

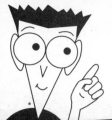

FOR DUMMIES®

The easy way to get more done and have more fun

and have more fun

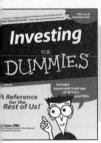
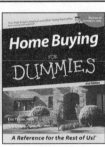
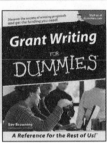
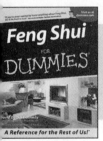
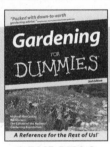
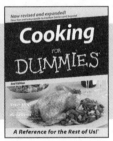
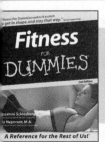
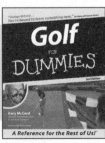
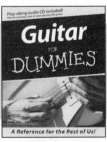
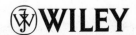

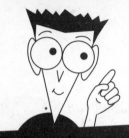

FOR DUMMIES®

A world of resources to help you grow

TRAVEL

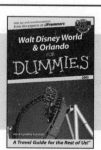

Italy For Dummies
0-7645-5453-0

Hawaii For Dummies
0-7645-5438-7

Walt Disney World & Orlando For Dummies
0-7645-5444-1

Also available:

America's National Parks For Dummies
(0-7645-6204-5)

Caribbean For Dummies
(0-7645-5445-X)

Cruise Vacations For Dummies 2003
(0-7645-5459-X)

Europe For Dummies
(0-7645-5456-5)

Ireland For Dummies
(0-7645-6199-5)

France For Dummies
(0-7645-6292-4)

Las Vegas For Dummies
(0-7645-5448-4)

London For Dummies
(0-7645-5416-6)

Mexico's Beach Resorts For Dummies
(0-7645-6262-2)

Paris For Dummies
(0-7645-5494-8)

RV Vacations For Dummie
(0-7645-5443-3)

EDUCATION & TEST PREPARATION

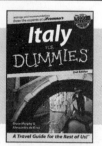

Spanish For Dummies
0-7645-5194-9

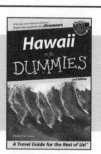

Algebra For Dummies
0-7645-5325-9

U.S. History For Dummies
0-7645-5249-X

Also available:

The ACT For Dummies
(0-7645-5210-4)

Chemistry For Dummies
(0-7645-5430-1)

English Grammar For Dummies
(0-7645-5322-4)

French For Dummies
(0-7645-5193-0)

GMAT For Dummies
(0-7645-5251-1)

Inglés Para Dummies
(0-7645-5427-1)

Italian For Dummies
(0-7645-5196-5)

Research Papers For Dumm
(0-7645-5426-3)

SAT I For Dummies
(0-7645-5472-7)

U.S. History For Dummies
(0-7645-5249-X)

World History For Dummie
(0-7645-5242-2)

HEALTH, SELF-HELP & SPIRITUALITY

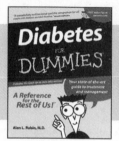

Diabetes For Dummies
0-7645-5154-X

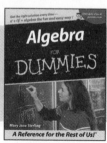

Sex For Dummies
0-7645-5302-X

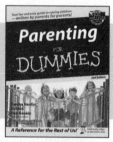

Parenting For Dummies
0-7645-5418-2

Also available:

The Bible For Dummies
(0-7645-5296-1)

Controlling Cholesterol For Dummies
(0-7645-5440-9)

Dating For Dummies
(0-7645-5072-1)

Dieting For Dummies
(0-7645-5126-4)

High Blood Pressure For Dummies
(0-7645-5424-7)

Judaism For Dummies
(0-7645-5299-6)

Menopause For Dummies
(0-7645-5458-1)

Nutrition For Dummies
(0-7645-5180-9)

Potty Training For Dummie
(0-7645-5417-4)

Pregnancy For Dummies
(0-7645-5074-8)

Rekindling Romance For Dummies
(0-7645-5303-8)

Religion For Dummies
(0-7645-5264-3)

Available wherever books are sold. Go to www.dummies.com or call 1-877-762-2974 to order direct

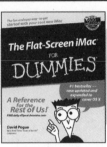
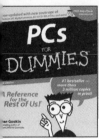
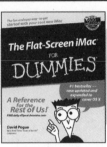
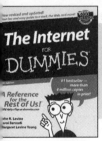
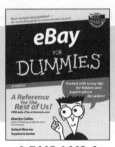
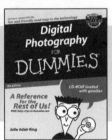

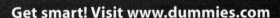

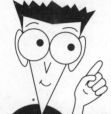
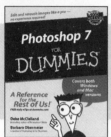
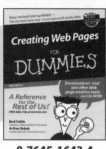
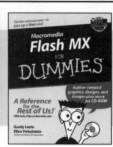
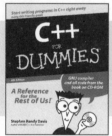
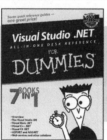
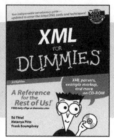
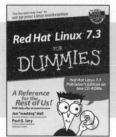
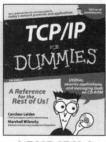
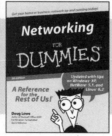
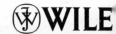